Workbook for

Pilbeam's Mechanical Ventilation:

Physiological and Clinical Applications

Fifth Edition

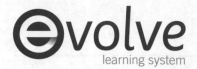
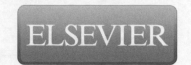
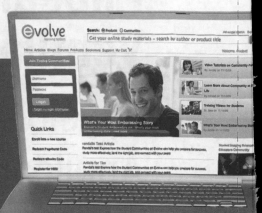

Workbook for

Pilbeam's Mechanical Ventilation:

Physiological and Clinical Applications

Fifth Edition

Sindee K. Karpel, MPA, RRT
Clinical Coordinator
Respiratory Care Program
Edison State College
Fort Myers, Florida

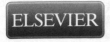
ELSEVIER

ELSEVIER
MOSBY

3251 Riverport Lane
St. Louis, Missouri 63043

WORKBOOK FOR PILBEAM'S MECHANICAL VENTILATION: ISBN: 978-0-323-07208-3
PHYSIOLOGICAL AND CLINICAL APPLICATIONS

Content Manager: Billie Sharp
Senior Content Development Specialist: Kathleen Sartori
Content Coordinator: Andrea Hunolt
Publishing Services Managers: Julie Eddy and Hemamalini Rajendrababu
Senior Project Managers: Andrea Campbell and Antony Prince
Designer: Karen Pauls

Printed in the United States of America

Last digit is the print number: 9   8   7   6   5   4   3   2   1

To my husband Larry and to my sons Brad and Jordan, for their unwavering support and encouragement, and to all my students—past, present and future—for providing me with the challenges that keep me learning.

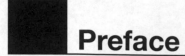

Preface

The goal of this workbook is to assist the respiratory care student in the mastery of the information presented in *Pilbeam's Mechanical Ventilation: Physiological and Clinical Applications,* Fifth Edition, by James M. Cairo.

Reading a textbook like this requires active participation, which is very different from the passive reading we do for pleasure. The reader should expect to read more slowly and carefully when the material is expected to be understood and remembered. Comprehension is not an automatic response to the movement of the eyes across a line of print. To actively participate in the reading process, the reader must focus attention on what information is needed from the material. Reading with a purpose (e.g., to answer questions) increases concentration, comprehension, retention, and interest in the subject matter.

I would like to suggest that the student use the text and workbook in the following manner:

First, preview or survey the text by reading the title, outline, objectives, and key terms. Remember: the learning objectives indicate what the author intends for the reader to know after finishing with the chapter. Skim the headings and subheadings. Read the Chapter summary. This highlights the structure of the chapter and emphasizes important concepts.

Next, turn the title into a question. The idea here is that asking a question focuses your reading on finding information that will answer the question. It makes reading a more active search for meaning. Use the review questions in the workbook to help you focus on important points in the chapter. Read carefully (in manageable chunks) to answer these questions. Note important details and relationships of ideas. The review questions in this workbook are based on the author's learning objectives for each chapter. Pay particular attention to the figures, boxes, tables, key points, case studies, and clinical scenarios because they are included to help learn the material.

Then review the textbook's Chapter Review Questions. Be able to answer all of the questions. This will ensure that highlighting or annotating the textbook is being done efficiently.

After this, answer the Critical Thinking Questions and the Case Study Questions in the Workbook. This will help with analysis and application-type questions seen on the board exams. The next step is to attempt the NBRC-type questions. Once this has been completed, test your critical vocabulary by trying the key terms crossword puzzle. ***All Answers for the Workbook are available through your Instructor via the Evolve website.***

Sindee K. Karpel, MPA, RRT

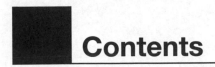

Contents

1 Basic Terms and Concepts of Mechanical Ventilation

LEARNING OBJECTIVES

Upon completion of this chapter the reader will be able to do the following:

1. Define *ventilation*, *external respiration*, and *internal respiration*.
2. Draw a graph showing how intrapleural and alveolar (intrapulmonary) pressures change during spontaneous ventilation and during a positive pressure breath.
3. Define the terms *transpulmonary pressure*, *transrespiratory pressure*, *transairway pressure*, *transthoracic pressure*, *elastance*, *compliance*, and *resistance*.
4. Provide the value for intra-alveolar pressure throughout inspiration and expiration during normal, quiet breathing.
5. Write the formulas for calculating compliance and resistance.
6. Explain how changes in lung compliance affect the peak pressure measured during inspiration with a mechanical ventilator.
7. Describe the airway conditions that can lead to increased resistance.
8. Calculate the airway resistance given the peak inspiratory pressure, a plateau pressure, and the flow rate.
9. From Figures 1-13 and 1-14 showing abnormal compliance or airway resistance, determine which lung unit will fill more quickly or with a greater volume.
10. Compare several time constants, and explain how different time constants will affect volume distribution during inspiration.
11. Give the percentage of passive filling (or emptying) for one, two, three, and five time constants.
12. Briefly discuss the principle of operation of negative pressure, positive pressure, and high-frequency mechanical ventilators.
13. Define *peak inspiratory pressure*, *baseline pressure*, *positive end-expiratory pressure* (PEEP), and *plateau pressure*.
14. Describe the measurement of plateau pressure.

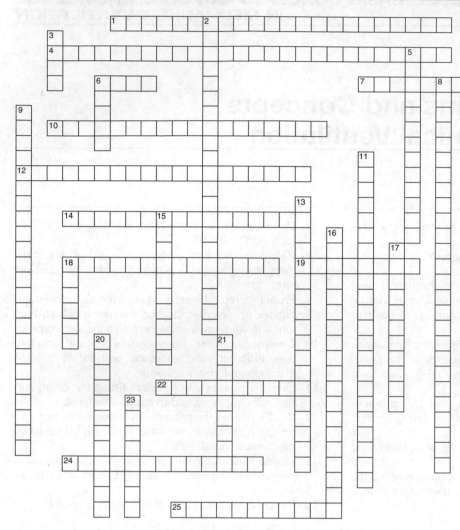

Across

1 An alternate term for pressure in the airways of the lungs (three words)
4 The total amount of gas remaining in the lungs after a resting expiration (three words)
6 Abbreviation for a form of ventilatory support characterized by rates up to 4000 breaths/minute
7 The pressure measurement when there is no gas flow
10 Pressure measured in the esophagus that is used to represent intrapleural pressure (two words)
12 The movement of oxygen into cells and the movement of carbon dioxide out of cells (two words)
14 The measurement of elastic forces that oppose lung inflation (two words)
18 Pressure in the airways of the lungs (two words)
19 Another term for auto-PEEP (hyphenated word)
22 The impedance of gas flow through the conductive airways
24 A deliberate increase in the ventilator's baseline pressure (two words)
25 The movement of gas molecules across a membrane.

Down

2 Pressure measured at the mouth (three words)
3 Abbreviation for ventilation using small pulses of pressurized gas at rates between 100 and 400 breaths/minute
5 A complication of positive pressure ventilation that causes an inadvertent buildup of positive pressure in the alveoli (two words)
6 Abbreviation for ventilation using lower than normal tidal volumes and respiratory rates between 60 and 100 breaths/minute
8 The pressure between the alveolus and the pleural space responsible for maintaining alveolar inflation (three words)
9 Another term for the highest pressure recorded at the end of inspiration (three words)
11 Airway communications between the lung and pleural space (two words)
13 The highest pressure recorded at the end of inspiration (three words)
15 The ease with which the lungs distend
16 The movement of oxygen into the bloodstream and carbon dioxide out of the bloodstream (two words)
17 The movement of air into the lungs for gas exchange and out of the lungs for carbon dioxide removal
18 A functional unit of the lung
20 A mathematical expression used to describe the filling and emptying of lung units (two words)
21 The tendency of the lungs to return to their original form after being stretched
23 The difference between an area of high pressure and low pressure

Chapter **1** **Basic Terms and Concepts of Mechanical Ventilation**

CHAPTER REVIEW QUESTIONS

1. Describe the difference between ventilation and respiration.

   _____

   _____

   _____

2. The movement of oxygen and carbon dioxide in and out of the alveolar capillaries is known as _____, whereas the movement of oxygen and carbon dioxide in and out of body tissues is called _____ .

3. Describe the conditions necessary for air to flow from Point A to Point B in Figure 1-1.

   Point A ⬭ **Point B**

   _____

   _____

4. The pressure in the potential space between the parietal and visceral pleura is known as _____. At the end of exhalation during spontaneous breathing this pressure is approximately _____ and at the end of inspiration is about _____ .

5. Use Figure 1-2 for this question.

   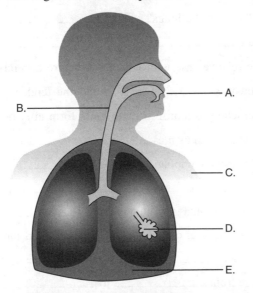

   a. Identify the pressures labeled *A* through *E*.

   _____

b. Name at least three additional terms for pressure *A*.

   1. _____

   2. _____

   3. _____

6. How is intrapleural pressure (P_{pl}) estimated?

   _____

   _____

   _____

7. The pressure gradient between airway pressure and alveolar pressure is known as _____. This pressure is responsible for the movement of air in the _____. This gradient is calculated by the formula _____ .

8. The pressure needed to expand or contract both the lungs and the chest wall at the same time is _____. This pressure gradient is calculated by the formula _____ .

9. The pressure that is responsible for maintaining alveolar inflation is known as _____ and is calculated by the formula _____ .

10. The pressure that is required for inflation of the lungs and airways during positive pressure ventilation is called _____ and is calculated by the formula _____ .

11. Use Figure 1-2 to answer questions a through d.

    a. What pressure gradient is represented by Point A to Point C? What is its function during breathing?

    _____

    _____

    b. What pressure gradient is represented by Point C to Point D? What is its function during breathing?

    _____

    _____

    c. What pressure gradient is represented by Point D to Point E? What is its function during breathing?

    _____

    _____

d. What pressure gradient is represented by Point B to Point D? What is its function during breathing?

_____

_____

12. On the graph in Figure 1-3, label the x and y axes; draw the changes in intra-alveolar pressure during a spontaneous breath, and label inspiration and expiration.

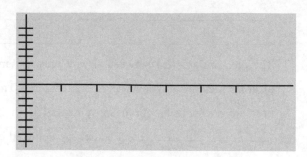

13. Describe how a negative pressure ventilator causes air to move into an individual's lungs.

_____

_____

_____

_____

14. List three advantages of using negative pressure ventilators.

1. _____

2. _____

3. _____

15. Calculate the transairway pressure when the mouth pressure (P_M) is +25 cm H_2O and the intra-alveolar pressure (P_{alv}) is +5 cm H_2O.

_____

16. Draw and label, on the graph in Figure 1-4, the changes in intrapulmonary pressure that occur during a positive pressure breath with a peak inspiratory pressure of 30 cm H_2O, a plateau pressure of 20 cm H_2O, PEEP of 5 cm H_2O, inspiratory time of 2 seconds, and expiratory time of 4 seconds.

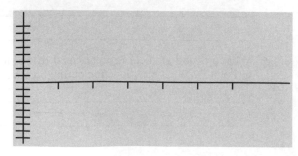

17. Draw and label, on the graph in Figure 1-5, the changes in intrapulmonary pressure that occur during a positive pressure breath with a peak inspiratory pressure of 45 cm H_2O, a plateau pressure of 25 cm H_2O, PEEP of 10 cm H_2O, inspiratory time of 1 second, and expiratory time of 2 seconds, followed by a spontaneous breath with the same baseline.

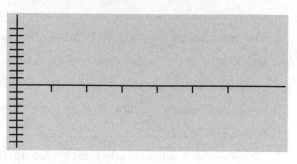

18. The highest pressure recorded at the end of inspiration is called _____

or _____.

19. The pressure at which expiration ends is called

_____.

20. When end expiratory pressure is above atmospheric pressure this is called _____.

21. The pressure required to overcome the elastic recoil of the lungs is known as _____ and is measured on a mechanically ventilated person by

_____.

22. What are the two types of forces that oppose inflation of the lungs? _____

and _____.

23. The relative ease with which a structure distends is known as _____ and the tendency of a structure to return to its original form after being stretched is known as _____.

24. Pulmonary compliance is defined as _____

_____

and the formula is written as _____.

25. Normally, total compliance of the lungs and thorax is about _____, but it can range from _____ to _____.

Chapter 1 Basic Terms and Concepts of Mechanical Ventilation

26. While being mechanically ventilated, the compliance value for a male with normal lungs is _____ and for a female with normal lungs is _____.

27. What is the formula to calculate static compliance?

_____

28. When more pressure is required to deliver a specific volume, what is happening to compliance?

_____

29. Calculate static compliance when plateau pressure is 27 cm H_2O, baseline pressure is 10 cm H_2O, and tidal volume is 750 mL.

_____

30. Calculate static compliance when plateau pressure is 35 cm H_2O, baseline pressure is 5 cm H_2O, and tidal volume is 575 mL.

_____

31. Calculate static compliance when plateau pressure is 18 cm H_2O, baseline pressure is 0 H_2O, and tidal volume is 650 mL.

_____

32. What happens to peak inspiratory pressures as the lungs become harder to ventilate? What happens to lung compliance?

_____

_____

33. Define *resistance*.

_____

_____

34. What is the formula for airway resistance (Raw)?

_____

35. What is the normal resistance range for flow rates of 0.5 L/sec?

_____

36. What lung disease causes both airway resistance and static compliance to increase?

_____

37. Calculate the transairway pressure (P_{ta}) when PIP is 27 cm H_2O and $P_{plateau}$ is 20 cm H_2O.

_____

_____

38. How much pressure is needed to overcome airway resistance when PIP is 30 cm H_2O and $P_{plateau}$ is 20 cm H_2O?

_____

39. What is the normal amount of pressure lost to airway resistance when a patient has a properly sized endotracheal tube?

_____

40. Calculate airway resistance for a ventilated patient with the following: PIP 48 cm H_2O, $P_{plateau}$ 30 cm H_2O, and a set flow rate of 40 L/minute.

_____

_____

_____

_____

41. Calculate airway resistance for a ventilated patient with the following: PIP 25 cm H_2O, $P_{plateau}$ 15 cm H_2O, and a set flow rate of 60 L/minute.

_____

_____

_____

42. Why are the characteristics of the lung not homogenous?

_____

_____

43. Compare the filling time and volume for a normal lung unit, a low compliance unit, and a unit with high airway resistance using the same driving pressure.

_____

_____

_____

_____

44. What factors contribute to resistance to breathing?

_____

_____

_____

_____

45. What clinical factors can increase airway resistance by decreasing the radius of the airways?

_____

_____

46. How many seconds will it take to allow 86% of the tidal volume to be exhaled when compliance is 25 mL/cm H_2O and resistance is 30 cm H_2O/L/sec?

_____

_____

47. Calculate the time constant for a mechanically ventilated patient when the tidal volume is 600 mL, PIP is 30 cm H_2O, $P_{plateau}$ is 24 cm H_2O, flow rate is 60 L/min, with no PEEP.

_____

_____

_____

_____

48. What percentage of passive filling occurs for 1, 2, 3, 4, and 5 time constants?

_____

_____

49. The time constant for patient #1 is 0.05 seconds; patient #2 is 3 seconds; and 0.5 seconds for patient #3. If the same filling pressure is used for each, which patient will receive the most volume during inspiration and why?

_____

_____

_____

50. Calculate the time constant for a compliance of 55 mL/cm H_2O and resistance of 6 cm H_2O/L/sec.

_____

_____

51. What is the inspiratory time setting to allow 95% volume emptying for a patient with the time constant calculated in question 50?

_____

_____

52. Why do patients with increased airway resistance develop air trapping with high set ventilator rates?

_____

_____

_____

53. Calculate the time constant for a mechanically ventilated patient when the tidal volume is 700 mL, PIP is 45 cm H_2O, $P_{plateau}$ is 18 cm H_2O, flow rate is 60 L/min, and PEEP 5 cm H_2O.

_____

_____

_____

_____

54. Which of the two lung units represented in Figure 1-6 will receive more volume given the same amount of time for inspiration? Explain your answer.

_____

_____

_____

55. Which of the two lung units represented in Figure 1-7 will fill more quickly? Explain your answer.

_____

_____

_____

6

1. When the PIP is 43 cm H_2O and the $P_{plateau}$ is 18 cm H_2O, how much pressure was required to overcome the resistance of the airways?

_____

_____

_____

2. What time constants would you expect for a patient with adult respiratory distress syndrome?

_____

_____

_____

3. Describe how emphysema causes lung units to have long time constants.

_____

_____

_____

4. What time constants would you expect for a 30-week (gestational age) premature infant?

_____

_____

_____

CASE STUDIES

Case Study 1

A respiratory therapist reviews the following information concerning an intubated patient being mechanically ventilated.

Time	PIP	$P_{plateau}$	Tidal Volume	Set Flow Rate	PEEP
0800	18 cm H_2O	10 cm H_2O	600 mL	45 L/min	5 cm H_2O
1000	24 cm H_2O	12 cm H_2O	600 mL	45 L/min	5 cm H_2O
1200	35 cm H_2O	11 cm H_2O	600 mL	45 L/min	5 cm H_2O

1. What is the transairway pressure at 0800, 1000, and 1200?

_____

_____

_____

2. Calculate the Raw for 0800, 1200, and 1200.

_____

_____

_____

3. Calculate the static compliance for 0800, 1000, and 1200.

_____

_____

_____

4. Calculate one time constant for 0800, 1000, and 1200.

_____

_____

_____

5. a. What caused the peak inspiratory pressure to rise between 0800 and 1200?

   b. What problems will this cause with ventilating the patient?

_____

_____

_____

Case Study 2

The following information is obtained from the flow sheet of an intubated patient being mechanically ventilated.

Time	PIP	$P_{plateau}$	Tidal Volume	Set Flow Rate	PEEP
1000	40 cm H_2O	28 cm H_2O	550 mL	40 L/min	0 cm H_2O
1200	47 cm H_2O	37 cm H_2O	550 mL	40 L/min	5 cm H_2O
1400	54 cm H_2O	43 cm H_2O	550 mL	40 L/min	7 cm H_2O
1600	45 cm H_2O	33 cm H_2O	450 mL	60 L/min	12 cm H_2O

1. Complete the table below.

Time	P_{ta}	Raw	C_{STAT}	Time Constant
1000				
1200				
1400				
1600				

2. What is the source of the rising peak inspiratory pressure between 1000 and 1400?

_____

3. What would be the minimum inspiratory time for this patient at 1600 hours?

_____

Chapter 1 **Basic Terms and Concepts of Mechanical Ventilation**

NBRC-STYLE QUESTIONS

1. Calculate the static effective compliance during the delivery of a ventilator breath with 650 mL with a $P_{plateau}$ of 28 cm H_2O.
   a. 0.04 cm H_2O/L
   b. 0.23 L/cm H_2O
   c. 23 mL/cm H_2O
   d. Not enough information is given

2. Calculate the airway resistance for a patient receiving mechanical ventilation with a set tidal volume of 825 mL and a peak flow setting of 50 L/min when the peak inspiratory pressure is 46 cm H_2O and the $P_{plateau}$ is 22 cm H_2O.
   a. 13.7 cm H_2O/L/sec
   b. 26.5 cm H_2O/L/sec
   c. 28.9 cm H_2O/L/sec
   d. 38.2 cm H_2O/L/sec

3. Calculate one time constant for the following data:
   Peak inspiratory pressure: 29 cm H_2O
   $P_{plateau}$: 23 cm H_2O
   Tidal volume: 600 mL
   PEEP: 5 cm H_2O
   Inspiratory flow rate: 45 L/min
   a. 0.017 seconds
   b. 0.021 seconds
   c. 0.21 seconds
   d. 0.27 seconds

4. The cause of a mechanically ventilated patient's peak inspiratory pressure to increase from 20 to 40 cm H_2O while the static compliance remains relatively unchanged is which of the following?
   a. Removed mucous plugs
   b. Increased airway resistance
   c. Tension pneumothorax
   d. Decreased elastance

5. An increase in peak inspiratory pressure and $P_{plateau}$ with a stable transairway pressure may be caused by which of the following?
   a. Acute respiratory distress syndrome
   b. Acute asthma exacerbation
   c. Retained secretions in the airways
   d. A too small endotracheal tube

6. Which of the following will occur when a patient's lung-thoracic compliance improves?
   1. $P_{plateau}$ decreases
   2. Peak inspiratory pressure decreases
   3. $P_{plateau}$ increases
   4. Transairway pressure increases
   a. 1 and 2 only
   b. 1 and 4 only
   c. 2 and 3 only
   d. 3 and 4 only

7. Over the course of several hours, a respiratory therapist has detected an increase in transairway pressure of a mechanically ventilated patient. The patient's $P_{plateau}$ has remained stable. Which of the following may be the cause of this increase?
   a. Improving lung-thoracic compliance
   b. Acute respiratory distress syndrome
   c. Fluid buildup in the peritoneal cavity
   d. Removal of airway secretions

8. A patient's transairway pressure is rising, while the $P_{plateau}$ is constant. Which of the following should be done to correct this problem?
   1. Administer a bronchodilator
   2. Place a large-bore needle in the third intercostal space.
   3. Measure auto-PEEP
   4. Suction airway secretions.
   a. 2 only
   b. 3 and 4 only
   c. 1 and 4 only
   d. 1 and 3 only

9. Calculate the static compliance for a patient who is being mechanically ventilated and has an exhaled tidal volume of 825 mL, $P_{plateau}$ of 47 cm H_2O, and PEEP of 8 cm H_2O.
   a. 15 mL/cm H_2O
   b. 18 mL/cm H_2O
   c. 21 mL/cm H_2O
   d. 47 mL/cm H_2O

10. Which of the following situations will demonstrate the highest airway resistance?
   a. PIP is 65 cm H_2O, $P_{plateau}$ is 55 cm H_2O, flow rate is 60 L/min
   b. PIP is 52 cm H_2O, $P_{plateau}$ is 18 cm H_2O, flow rate is 45 L/min
   c. PIP is 45 cm H_2O, $P_{plateau}$ is 30 cm H_2O, flow rate is 50 L/min
   d. PIP is 30 cm H_2O, $P_{plateau}$ is 10 cm H_2O, flow rate is 40 L/min

Chapter 1 Basic Terms and Concepts of Mechanical Ventilation

2 How Ventilators Work

LEARNING OBJECTIVES

Upon completion of this chapter the reader will be able to do the following:

1. List the basic types of power sources used for mechanical ventilators.
2. Give examples of ventilators that use an electrical power source and a pneumatic power source.
3. Explain the difference in function between positive and negative pressure ventilators.
4. Distinguish between a closed-loop and an open-loop system.
5. Define *user interface*.
6. Describe a ventilator's internal and external pneumatic circuits.
7. Discuss the difference between a single-circuit and a double-circuit ventilator.
8. Identify the components of an external circuit (patient circuit).
9. Explain the function of an externally mounted exhalation valve.
10. Compare the functions of the three different types of volume displacement drive mechanisms.
11. Describe the function of the proportional solenoid valve.

11

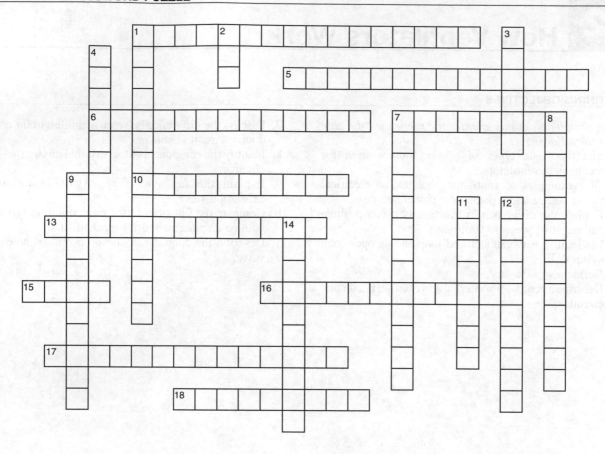

Across

1 A pathway of tubes within the ventilator is an internal (two words) _____
5 A single chip made of integrated circuits
6 Another name for the control panel (two words)
7 A pneumatic valve that uses an electromagnetic field and is controlled by a microprocessor
10 A device for which the internal volume can be changed
13 What's inside the black box
15 A type of controller
16 A stepper motor that controls a hinged clamp device (two words)
17 The mechanical device that causes gas to flow to the patient (two words)
18 Uses 50 psi as a power source

Down

1 Connects to the patient (two words)
2 A ventilator mode where the operator sets a minimum minute ventilation (abbreviation)
3 A mechanism to change internal volume
4 A type of controller
7 From ventilator directly to patient type ventilator (two words)
8 This type of ventilator has two internal pneumatic circuits (two words)
9 A type of valve that controls gas flow (two words)
11 An unintelligent system (two words)
12 An intelligent system (two words)
14 Uses AC or DC as a power source

CHAPTER REVIEW QUESTIONS

1. Name the three types of power sources used by ventilators that provide energy to perform the work of ventilating the patient.

   a. _____

   b. _____

   c. _____

2. What specific power source does each of the following ventilators use?

   Bird Mark 7 _____

   Intermed Bear 33 Homecare Ventilator _____

   _____

   Lifecare PLV-102 _____

   Servo^i _____

   LTV 800, 900, and 1000 _____

   Bio-Med MVP-10 _____

3. Describe an open loop system.

   _____

   _____

4. Describe a closed loop system.

   _____

   _____

5. How do ventilators cause air to move into the lungs?

   _____

6. Explain the difference in function between positive- and negative-pressure ventilators.

   _____

   _____

   _____

   _____

7. The place on the ventilator where the operator inputs the desired ventilator parameters is known as the

   _____.

8. Inside a ventilator, gas flow passes through what type of circuit?

   _____

9. After exiting the ventilator, gas flow passes through

   the _____ on

   its way to the patient.

10. The gas flow from the ventilator's power source goes directly to the patient. This is known as what type of internal pneumatic circuit? _____

    _____

11. The primary power source of a ventilator generates a gas flow that compresses another mechanism, such as a bellows or bag. The gas within this mechanism goes to the patient. This is a description of what type of internal pneumatic circuit?

    _____

    _____

12. List the four basic elements of a patient circuit.

    a. _____

    b. _____

    c. _____

    d. _____

13. Identify the labeled parts of the ventilator circuit shown in Figure 2-1.

    a. _____

    b. _____

    c. _____

    d. _____

14. Explain how an external exhalation valve operates.

    _____

    _____

    _____

    _____

    _____

15. Name two types of flow control valves available on current ventilators.

    a. _____

    b. _____

16. Describe how each of the flow control valves operates.

_____

_____

_____

_____

_____

_____

17. The internal hardware that converts electrical or pneumatic energy to a system that provides a breath to a patient is called the _____.

18. Name four types of compressors that are used in ventilators.

a. _____

b. _____

c. _____

d. _____

19. Describe how a spring-loaded bellows functions.

_____

_____

20. Describe how a linear drive piston functions.

_____

_____

21. Describe how a rotary drive piston functions.

_____

_____

_____

_____

22. The ICU ventilators used today have what type of internal functions?

_____

_____

23. What type of ventilator uses the Coanda effect as its internal control system?

_____

CRITICAL THINKING QUESTIONS

1. A patient being ventilated in the SIMV mode becomes apneic. Explain how both closed and open loop systems might respond to this occurrence.

_____

_____

_____

2. If the exhalation valve malfunctions, what happens to the inspiratory gas flow?

_____

_____

3. What type of ventilator could be used during an MRI procedure?

_____

_____

CASE STUDIES

Case Study 1

A patient receiving mechanical ventilation needs to be transported to another medical center for treatment. What type of power source would be appropriate for use during patient transport?

_____

_____

Case Study 2

While being mechanically ventilated in a mode that allows spontaneous breathing, a patient becomes apneic. The ventilator automatically alarms and switches to full ventilatory support. Is this an open or closed loop system? Explain.

_____

_____

_____

NBRC-STYLE QUESTIONS

1. The power used by a mechanical ventilator to perform the work of ventilating the patient is known as which of the following?
   a. Force
   b. Pressure
   c. Input power
   d. Output power

2. Which of the following statement(s) is (are) true concerning combined power ventilators?
   1. They must have an electrical power source and two 50-psi gas sources.
   2. They often have RAM and ROM for data and preprogrammed modes.
   3. The electrical power provides the energy to deliver the breath.
   4. The pneumatic power controls the internal function of the machine.
   a. 2 only
   b. 1 and 3 only
   c. 3 and 4 only
   d. 1, 2, and 4 only

3. The internal circuit of a ventilator has the gas go directly from its power source to the patient. This is known as which of the following?
   a. External circuit
   b. Internal circuit
   c. Single circuit
   d. Double circuit

4. One of the functions of the exhalation valve is to do which of the following?
   a. Regulate pressure
   b. Ensure adequate humidification
   c. Ensure gas delivery on inspiration
   d. Determine the patient's tidal volume

5. A closed loop system is being used to guarantee minute ventilation to a patient. The minute volume delivered to the patient differs significantly from the set minute volume. The ventilator will do which of the following?
   a. Alarm and shut off
   b. Switch to 100% oxygen
   c. Double the minute volume
   d. Alter the volume delivered

6. The mechanical device that causes gas to flow to the patient is known as which of the following?
   a. Drive mechanism
   b. Power transmission
   c. Exhalation valve
   d. Solenoid valve

7. Volume displacement devices include which of the following?
   1. Pistons
   2. Stepper motors
   3. Concertina bags
   4. Proportional solenoids
   a. 1 and 4 only
   b. 1 and 3 only
   c. 2 and 3 only
   d. 2 and 4 only

8. The flow control valve that uses an electromagnetic field is which of the following?
   a. Digital valve
   b. Stepper motor
   c. Solenoid valve
   d. Rotating blade

9. Which type of ventilator uses the wall attachment phenomenon or Coanda effect as its basic component?
   a. Fluidic ventilator
   b. Electrically powered ventilator
   c. Pneumatically powered ventilator
   d. Microprocessor controlled ventilator

10. The volume displacement device that creates a sinusoidal flow wave pattern during inspiration is which of the following?
    a. Spring-loaded bellows
    b. Linear drive piston
    c. Rotary drive piston
    d. Concertina bag

5 Selecting the Ventilator and the Mode

LEARNING OBJECTIVES

Upon completion of this chapter the reader will be able to do the following:

1. Select an appropriate mechanical ventilation mode based on findings derived from a patient's history and physical assessment.
2. Describe two methods of delivering noninvasive positive-pressure ventilation (NIV).
3. Compare the advantages and disadvantages of volume-controlled and pressure-controlled ventilation.
4. Explain the differences in function between continuous mandatory ventilation, synchronized intermittent mandatory ventilation, and spontaneous ventilation.
5. Use the terms *trigger, cycle,* and *limit* to define volume-targeted continuous mandatory ventilation,

pressure-targeted continuous mandatory ventilation, assist/control ventilation, volume-targeted synchronized intermittent mandatory ventilation, pressure-targeted synchronized intermittent mandatory ventilation, and pressure support ventilation.
6. Define each of the following terms: *pressure augmentation, pressure-regulated volume control, volume support, mandatory minute ventilation, airway pressure release ventilation, bilevel positive airway pressure,* and *proportional assist ventilation.*
7. Give examples of the types of patients who would benefit most from each mode of ventilation.

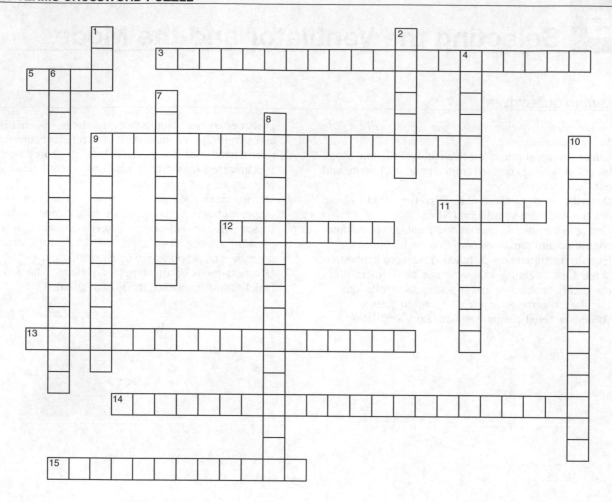

Across

3 Overventilation in the CMV mode will cause this (two words)
5 A mode of ventilation that uses two levels of CPAP (abbreviation)
9 When the patient controls the timing and the tidal volume (two words)
11 Inverse ventilation with pressure control (abbreviation)
12 A type of control variable
13 Mode of ventilation with only time-triggered breaths (two words)
14 The ventilator supplies all the energy necessary to maintain alveolar ventilation (three words)
15 Occurs when the patient and the ventilator are not working together

Down

1 Mode of ventilation where all breaths are mandatory and can be volume- or pressure-targeted (abbreviation)
2 Type of ventilatory support where patient is participating in the WOB
4 Patient-triggered volume or pressure-targeted ventilation (hyphenated word)
6 A mode that supports the spontaneously breathing patient to help reduce WOB (two words)
7 Type of breath where the timing and/or the tidal volume is controlled by the ventilator
8 Guarantees a specific volume delivery (two words)
9 The ventilator setting used to determine the ventilator response to the patient's inspiratory effort
10 A cross between mandatory and spontaneous breaths

CHAPTER REVIEW QUESTIONS

1. Name seven criteria that ventilator selection is based upon.

   a. _____

   b. _____

   c. _____

   d. _____

   e. _____

   f. _____

   g. _____

2. Match the appropriate ventilation support type with the appropriate ventilator connection or interface (there may be more than one answer):

   _____ Negative pressure ventilation   A. Oral endotracheal tube

   _____ Continuous positive airway pressure   B. Nasal mask

   _____ Positive pressure ventilation   C. Face mask

   _____ Noninvasive positive pressure ventilation   D. Chest cuirass

       E. Tracheostomy tube

3. Continuous positive airway pressure is commonly used in the hospital environment for _____ and in the home setting for treating _____.

4. Acute-on-chronic respiratory failure is most often treated with which type of NIV? _____

   _____.

5. What type of ventilation reduces the requirements for heavy patient sedation?

   _____

6. Define *full ventilatory support* and *partial ventilatory support*.

   _____

   _____

   _____

7. The minimum rate setting to be considered full ventilatory support is _____.

8. Partial ventilatory support is any amount of mechanical ventilation with set machine rates that are less than _____.

9. What type of ventilatory support should be used when the patient has acute ventilatory failure due to ventilatory muscle fatigue or a high work of breathing? Why?

   _____

   _____

   _____

10. Choose the type of breath delivery (mandatory breath, spontaneous breath or assisted breath) that matches the description:

    a. Flow-triggered, pressure-targeted, time-cycled:

       _____.

    b. Time-triggered, volume-targeted, volume-cycled:

       _____.

    c. Pressure-triggered, pressure-targeted, time-cycled:

       _____.

    d. Flow-triggered, pressure-triggered, flow-cycled:

       _____.

11. What is the main advantage of volume ventilation?

    _____

    _____

    _____

12. During volume ventilation a patient develops bronchospasm. What will happen to (a) the peak inspiratory pressure? Why? What will happen to (b) the amount of volume delivered to the patient? Why?

    a. _____

       _____

    b. _____

       _____

13. A patient having bronchospasm receives an adrenergic bronchodilator. The peak inspiratory pressure is expected to _____ because the patient's lung condition has improved.

14. What are the advantages and disadvantages of using NIV in acute respiratory failure?

    _____

    _____

    _____

15. When a patient's lung compliance worsens, during volume ventilation, what will happen to peak inspiratory pressure? What will happen to alveolar pressure?

_____

_____

16. What may result when sensitivity is set inappropriately insensitive?

_____

_____

17. When targeting pressure as the control variable, what will vary with changing lung characteristics?

_____

18. When a patient's lung compliance worsens, during pressure targeted ventilation, what will happen to volume delivery? _____ This may lead to alveolar _____ (hyperventilation; hypoventilation). When a patient's lung condition improves, _____ (more; less) volume is delivered.

19. Complete the following table:

Type of Ventilation	Advantages	Disadvantages
Volume Ventilation	_____	_____
	_____	_____
	_____	_____
	_____	_____
	_____	_____
	_____	_____
	_____	_____
	_____	_____
	_____	_____
	_____	_____
Pressure Ventilation	_____	_____
	_____	_____
	_____	_____
	_____	_____
	_____	_____
	_____	_____
	_____	_____
	_____	_____

20. Which type of ventilation demonstrates more benefit for spontaneously breathing patients when used with a descending flow pattern?

_____

21. Name the three breath delivery techniques.

a. _____

b. _____

c. _____

22. Continuous mandatory ventilation (CMV), is also known as:

a. _____

b. _____

c. _____

23. What trigger is used when a ventilator is in the control mode?

_____

24. For what types of patients is controlled ventilation appropriate?

_____

_____

_____

25. What patient situations may call for the use of paralysis with medications and/or sedation?

_____

_____

_____

26. What two patient situations may benefit from deliberate (iatrogenic) hyperventilation? Why?

a. _____

b. _____

27. What happens when the ventilator is made totally insensitive to patient effort?

_____

_____

28. What three triggers may begin inspiration in the assist-control mode?

a. _____

b. _____

c. _____

29. What can happen to a patient's acid-base status if the patient's ventilatory drive increases while receiving mechanical ventilation in the assist-control (CMV) mode?

_____

_____

30. When inspiration is active in VC-CMV and the set gas flow is inadequate, how much of the work of inspiration is done by the patient?

_____

_____

31. What are the control variables in PC-CMV?

_____

_____

32. A safety mechanism to avoid excessive system pressure is the _____ and is set at about _____ above the set PCV and will cause _____ to end when reached.

33. What ventilator mode should be used when it is more important to guard against increasing pressures than it is to guarantee a tidal volume?

_____

_____

34. When is the use of pressure control inverse ratio ventilation (PCIRV) appropriate?

_____

_____

35. How does IMV differ from CMV?

_____

_____

_____

36. How does SIMV differ from IMV?

_____

_____

_____

Chapter 5   Selecting the Ventilator and the Mode

37. What are the three basic means of providing support for continuous spontaneous breathing?

    a. _____

    b. _____

    c. _____

38. What can be used to reduce the WOB for spontaneous breaths during ventilation in SIMV mode? _____

39. What are the advantages and risks/disadvantages of using the assist-control mode?

    _____

    _____

    _____

40. What are the advantages and risks/disadvantages of using the IMV/SIMV mode?

    _____

    _____

    _____

41. What can cause dyssynchrony during pressure support ventilation?

    _____

42. What are the advantages and disadvantages of having an intubated patient breathe spontaneously through a ventilator circuit?

    _____

    _____

43. What type of patient would be appropriate for pressure-support ventilation (PSV)?

    _____

    _____

44. What ventilator parameters are set by the operator in the PSV mode?

    _____

45. In PSV what determines the patient tidal volume?

    _____

    _____

46. What situation will cause a mechanical ventilator in the PSV mode to time cycle?

    _____

47. What situation will cause a mechanical ventilator in the PSV mode to pressure cycle?

    _____

48. What are the three basic functions of PSV?

    a. _____

    b. _____

    c. _____

49. The time required for the ventilator to rise to the set pressure at the beginning of inspiration is known as

    _____ .

50. A very high flow setting in PSV may cause inspiration to _____ .

51. PSV ends inspiration by _____ cycling.

52. What are the triggers for bi-level pressure assist?

    _____

53. What variables end inspiration in the bi-level pressure assist mode?

    _____

54. Varying tidal volume delivery during pressure ventilation can be avoided by using closed-loop techniques such as _____ , _____ , and _____ .

55. How does P_{aug} work?

    _____

    _____

56. In P_{aug}, if the set volume is achieved prior to flow-cycling, what happens to the breath?

    _____

57. In P_{aug}, if the set volume is not reached before flow drops to the set level, how will the ventilator respond?

    _____

    _____

58. Under what condition can a patient receive more volume than set in P_{aug}?

    _____

    _____

59. Describe pressure regulated volume control (PRVC) in terms of trigger, limit, and cycle.

_____

60. At what pressure will a ventilator alarm while in the PRVC mode with the upper pressure limit set at 40 cm H_2O and a volume of 600 mL?

_____

_____

61. Describe volume support (VS) in terms of trigger, limit, and cycle.

_____

62. What is the difference between PRVC and VS?

_____

_____

_____

63. The method of ventilation that provides whatever part of the $\dot{V}_E$ that the patient is not able to accomplish is known as _____.

64. In MVV, what alarms must be set to protect against the problem of rapid shallow breathing?

_____

_____

65. The mode of ventilation that requires two levels of CPAP and allows the patient to breathe spontaneously at both levels is known as

_____.

66. The optimum duration of the release time for the mode mentioned in Question 65 is a function of the

_____ of the respiratory system.

67. APRV was originally intended to ventilate patients with _____.

68. With proportional assist ventilation (PAV), what variables are proportional to the patient's spontaneous effort?

_____

69. In the PAV mode what two factors determine the amount of pressure produced by the ventilator?

a. _____

b. _____

70. What are the advantages and disadvantages of PAV?

_____

_____

_____

_____

CRITICAL THINKING QUESTIONS

1. A patient is waking up following surgery and is currently receiving mechanical ventilation in the PC-CMV mode. During rounds the respiratory therapist observes the patient's use of accessory muscles, diaphoresis, patient-ventilator asynchrony, and no assisted breaths. What is the most probable source of this patient's clinical appearance? How can this be corrected?

_____

_____

_____

_____

2. If a patient's ventilatory drive increases during the use of VC-CMV, what changes will occur to the patient's acid-base balance? What can be done to regulate this?

_____

_____

_____

3. Which mode of ventilation would a home care patient with central sleep apnea benefit from and why?

_____

_____

_____

_____

4. Match the type of patient with the ventilator mode most likely to benefit the patient.

A patient with the following:

_____ (1) Intubated with quadriplegia from a spinal cord injury

_____ (2) Intubated with acute respiratory distress syndrome

_____ (3) Obstructive sleep apnea at home

_____ (4) Intubated with spontaneous breathing with acute lung injury

_____ (5) Intubated with consistent spontaneous respiratory pattern

_____ (6) Non-intubated spontaneously breathing with refractory hypoxemia

_____ (7) Intubated with drug overdose

Would benefit from this ventilator mode:

a. Nasal mask CPAP
b. CPAP through ventilator
c. Pressure support
d. VC-CMV
e. PC-CMV with PEEP

CASE STUDIES

Case Study 1

In the intensive care unit a respiratory therapist approaches a patient receiving mechanical ventilation. The ventilator monitor shows the following scalar.

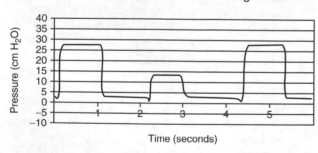

1. What mode of ventilation is the ventilator set to deliver?

_____

2. What is the inspiratory time for the mechanical breaths?

_____

3. What is the ventilator expiratory time?

_____

Case Study 2

A 6-foot 3-inch male motor vehicle accident (MVA) victim arrives in the ED with chest and facial injuries. Due to the nature of the facial injuries, he is intubated with a size 7 endotracheal tube. Following resuscitative measures he is transferred to the intensive care unit.

1. What type of ventilator support would this patient require initially?

_____

2. What ventilator mode would be appropriate when this patient wakes, has the desire to breathe spontaneously, and has a PaO_2 of 58 mm Hg with the F_IO_2 set at 50%?

_____

Case Study 3

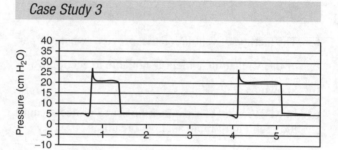

1. What mode of ventilation does Figure 5-2 represent?

_____

2. Identify the problem with this pressure tracing.

_____

3. What can be done to remedy the identified problem?

_____

NBRC–STYLE QUESTIONS

1. When switching from the CMV mode to the SIMV mode to facilitate weaning from mechanical ventilation, which of the following could be used, in addition to SIMV, to assist in this process?
   a. PCV
   b. PSV
   c. PAV
   d. APRV

2. A post-thoracic surgery patient currently receiving mechanical ventilation on VC-CMV with 60% oxygen has the following ABGs: pH 7.45, $PaCO_2$ 36 mm Hg, PaO_2 68 mm Hg. The patient's peak inspiratory pressures are averaging 55 cm H_2O. The ventilator mode that is most appropriate at this time is which of the following?
   a. PSV
   b. VC-SIMV with PEEP
   c. PC-CMV with PEEP
   d. MMV

3. A 38-year-old female suffered a deceleration injury in an MVA. She is alert and oriented but in respiratory distress. A piece of the patient's right anterior chest wall is moving in a paradoxical motion. Breath sounds are decreased on the right and the trachea is midline. ABG data reveals pH 7.48, $PaCO_2$ 31 mm Hg, PaO_2 63 mm Hg. The respiratory therapist should recommend which of the following for this patient at this time?
   a. Mask CPAP with supplemental oxygen
   b. Intubate and use VC-CMV with PEEP
   c. NIPPV with supplemental oxygen
   d. Intubate and use PCIRV

4. The physician requests that the respiratory therapist make a recommendation for a patient with post-polio complaints of increasing daytime weakness. Her vital capacity is 12 mL/kg and MIP is −32 cm H_2O. Her ABG on room air reveals pH 7.38, $PaCO_2$ 46 mm Hg, PaO_2 74 mm Hg. The respiratory therapist should suggest which of the following?
   a. Tracheostomy with PSV
   b. Tracheostomy with VC-CMV
   c. Bi-level PAP via nose mask at night
   d. Mask CPAP with supplemental oxygen

5. During a pressure triggered breath in VC-CMV the pressure-time curve on the graphic display does not rise smoothly and appears to be somewhat concave in appearance. This indicates which of the following?
   a. Flow rate is inadequate
   b. Rise time is set too slow
   c. Overshoot on the pressure
   d. Inspiratory time is too short

6. Every breath from the ventilator is time- or patient-triggered, pressure-targeted (limited), and time-cycled. This describes which of the following ventilator modes?
   a. P_{Aug}
   b. APRV
   c. PC-CMV
   d. VC-SIMV

7. Pressure augmentation (P_{Aug}) may be beneficial for mechanically ventilated patients with which of the following?
   1. Non-cardiogenic pulmonary edema
   2. Acute respiratory distress syndrome
   3. Postoperative upper abdominal surgery
   4. Receiving heavy sedation and paralyzing agents
   a. 1 and 2 only
   b. 1 and 3 only
   c. 2 and 4 only
   d. 3 and 4 only

8. The ventilator mode that allows the patient to breathe spontaneously at two levels of positive pressure is known as which of the following?
   a. BiPAP®
   b. P_{Aug}
   c. PRVC
   d. APRV

9. A patient is intubated and on PSV. The respiratory therapist notices that inspiratory time has increased from 1 second to 2 seconds consistently on every breath since last ventilator rounds. What action should the respiratory therapist take first?
   a. Change to the SIMV mode
   b. Check the ET tube cuff pressure
   c. Increase the inspiratory flow setting
   d. Suction and lavage the patient's airway

10. When lung compliance decreases while a patient is receiving mechanical ventilation with PC-CMV which of the following will occur?
   a. Peak pressure will increase
   b. Peak pressure will decrease
   c. Tidal volume will increase
   d. Tidal volume will decrease

6 Initial Ventilator Settings

LEARNING OBJECTIVES

Upon completion of this chapter the reader will be able to do the following:

1. Calculate tubing compliance.
2. Determine volume loss due to tubing compliance.
3. Calculate minute ventilation given a patient's rate and tidal volume.
4. Calculate total cycle time, inspiratory time, expiratory time, flow in L/sec, and inspiratory to expiratory ratios given the necessary patient data.
5. Select an appropriate flow rate and pattern.
6. Calculate initial minute ventilation, tidal volume, and rate for a patient placed on VC-CMV based on the patient's sex, height, and ideal body weight.
7. Identify the source of the problem when an inspiratory pause cannot be measured.
8. Choose an appropriate initial mode of mechanical ventilation and determine V_E, tidal volume, respiratory frequency, and positive end-expiratory pressure settings based on the patient's lung pathology, body temperature, metabolic rate, altitude, and acid-base balance.
9. Evaluate the response in peak inspiratory pressure and plateau pressure when the flow waveform is changed.
10. Recommend the selection and initial settings for the various modes of pressure ventilation, including bilevel positive airway pressure, pressure-supported ventilation, pressure-controlled ventilation, and Servo-controlled (dual modes) ventilation.
11. Identify a problem in pressure support ventilation from a pressure-time graph.
12. Measure plateau pressure using pressure-time and flow-time waveforms during pressure-controlled mechanical ventilation.
13. List the possible causes for a change in pressure during pressure-regulated volume control.
14. Identify the mode of ventilation based on the trigger, target, and cycle criteria.

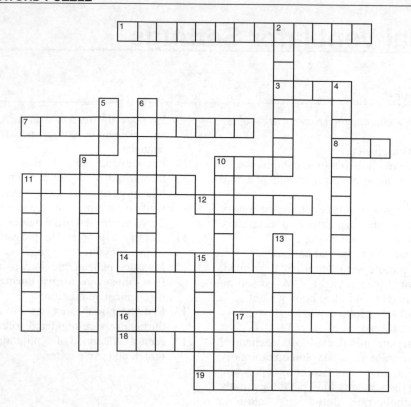

Across

1 Too much pressure in the alveoli can cause this
3 The abbreviation for a pressure-limited, time-cycled mode that uses the set tidal volume as a feedback control
7 Airway resistance multiplied by lung compliance is one _____ (two words)
8 The type of ventilation used to augment spontaneous breathing in patients with artificial airways (abbreviation)
10 The name of the type of flow waveform that represents the tapered flow at the end of inspiratory phase
11 A type of flow pattern created by a progressive increase in flow during inspiration
12 The chart used to determine BSA
14 The type of volume that is lost in the patient circuit
17 The Drager 500 calls its volume support by this name
18 The type of ventilator that has no flow waveform selector or peak flow control
19 The type of flow waveform that occurs naturally in pressure ventilation

Down

2 On the Hamiton G5 ventilator, PRVC is called _____ pressure ventilation
4 To calculate how much volume is lost in the patient circuit tubing, _____ must be known
5 One entire breathing cycle (abbreviation)
6 The type of pause used to measure plateau pressure
9 Adding tubing to the patient's endotracheal tube will add this type of dead space
10 A constant flow pattern produces this type of flow waveform
11 Air trapping is measured as this
13 The amount of inspiratory time required for the ventilator to reach the set pressure at the beginning of inspiration (two words)
15 The nomogram used to obtain ventilator settings
16 A purely spontaneous mode in which the operator sets the ventilator sensitivity, tidal volume, and upper pressure limit (abbreviation)

1. To meet the oxygen and carbon dioxide transport requirements, mechanical ventilation must support the patient's

   _____.

2. Name eight parameters that must be considered for volume ventilation setup.

   a. _____   e. _____

   b. _____   f. _____

   c. _____   g. _____

   d. _____   h. _____

3. Normal total body oxygen consumption is approximately _____ and carbon dioxide

   production is approximately _____.

Questions 4–6 refer to Figure 6-1.

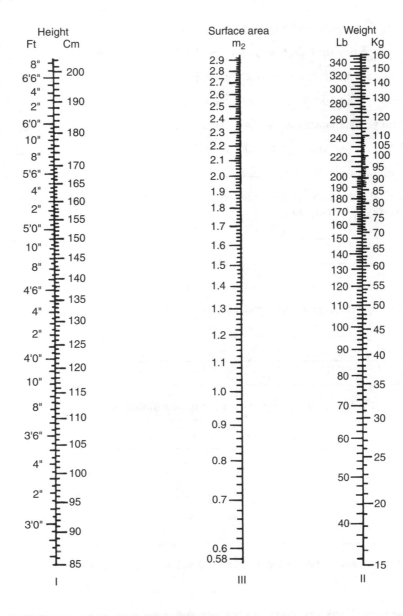

Chapter **6** **Initial Ventilator Settings**

4. Find the body surface area for a person who weighs 200 pounds and is 6 feet 2 inches tall.

_____

5. Find the body surface area for a person who weighs 75 kilograms and is 155 centimeters tall.

_____

6. Find the body surface area for a person who weighs 178 pounds and is 5 feet 7 inches tall.

_____

Questions 7–10: Calculate minute ventilation for the following individuals:

Question	Gender	BSA	Body Temp.	Comment	Minute Ventilation
7.	F	$1.6\,m^2$	39° C	N/A	_____
8.	M	$2.8\,m^2$	37° C	6000 ft above sea level	_____
9.	M	$2.3\,m^2$	101° F	N/A	_____
10.	F	$1.9\,m^2$	98.6° F	Metabolic acidosis	_____

11. The initial tidal volume setting for adults should be within what range? _____

12. The initial tidal volume setting for infants and children should be within what range? _____

13. The estimated V_T range for a 5 foot 4 inches tall female is _____

14. The estimated V_T range for a 6 foot 2 inches tall male is _____

15. What is the normal range for spontaneous V_T in a human? _____

16. What is the normal range for spontaneous breathing rate in a human? _____

17. The normal minute ventilation is about _____.

18. Calculate the initial tidal volume, respiratory rate, and minute ventilation for a 5 foot 2 inches tall female who has just arrived in the postoperative care unit.

_____

_____

_____

19. Calculate the initial tidal volume, respiratory rate, and minute ventilation for a 71 inches tall male with COPD.

_____

_____

_____

20. Calculate the initial tidal volume, respiratory rate, and minute ventilation for a 69 inches tall male with pulmonary fibrosis.

_____

_____

_____

21. If the measured tidal volume is 300 mL and the static pressure is 110 cm H_2O, the tubing compliance is how much?

_____

22. Calculate the tubing compliance when the measured tidal volume is 210 mL and the static pressure is 115 cm H_2O.

_____

23. The tubing compliance for a patient circuit is $2.5\,mL/cm\,H_2O$. Calculate the volume lost when the estimated V_T is $300\,mL$ and the peak inspiratory pressure to deliver each breath is approximately $28\,cm\,H_2O$.

_____

24. Calculate the actual delivered tidal volume when the tubing compliance is $1.8\,mL/cm\,H_2O$ and the set tidal volume is $450\,mL$ and the peak pressure is $30\,cm\,H_2O$.

_____

_____

25. For ventilators that do not compensate for tubing compliance, what should the respiratory therapist do?

_____

26. Calculate and fill in the missing information:

Tidal Volume	Respiratory Rate	Minute Ventilation
a. 750 mL	12 b/m	_____
b. 580 mL	10 b/m	_____
c. _____	15 b/m	6.9 L/min
d. _____	20 b/m	8.3 L/min
e. 460 mL	_____	5.2 L/min
f. 660 mL	_____	9.5 L/min

27. Calculate the total cycle time (TCT). TCT for the following frequencies (ie: rate setting):

a. 30 b/m _____

b. 15 b/m _____

c. 12 b/m _____

d. 10 b/m _____

28. Use the corresponding frequencies in Question 27 to calculate the T_E given the following T_I:

a. $T_I = 1$ second _____

b. $T_I = 0.75$ second _____

c. $T_I = 1.25$ seconds _____

d. $T_I = 2$ seconds _____

29. Use the corresponding information from Question 28 to reduce the I:E ratio to its simplest form:

a. _____

b. _____

c. _____

d. _____

30. Calculate T_I, T_E, and TCT given a 1:3 ratio and rate = 12 b/m.

_____

_____

_____

Chapter **6** **Initial Ventilator Settings**

31. Calculate T_I, T_E, and TCT given a 1:2 ratio and rate = 25 b/m.

_____

_____

32. Calculate V_T given T_I = 1 second and flow 50 L/min.

_____

_____

33. Calculate T_I given V_T = 700 mL and flow 50 L/min.

_____

_____

34. Increasing the set flow rate while ventilating an apneic patient with CMV will cause the T_I to _____, the PIP to _____, and the gas distribution to _____.

35. Explain what happens to T_I, T_E, PIP, and gas distribution when slower flow rates are used.

_____

_____

_____

36. What are the guidelines for setting inspiratory time, I:E ratio, and flow rates?

_____

37. The type of flow waveform pattern created by pressure ventilation is the _____.

38. The flow waveform that creates the highest PIP during volume ventilation, when Raw is elevated, is the _____.

39. The flow waveform(s) most appropriate for normal lungs is (are) _____.

40. Why is the descending flow pattern beneficial for patients with hypoxemia and low lung compliance?

_____

_____

41. For what is inspiratory pause used most frequently?

_____

42. The respiratory therapist attempts to measure plateau pressure by adding a 1-second inspiratory pause. The set VC-CMV rate is 12, the current rate is 20, and the plateau pressure is unattainable. What is the cause of this problem?

_____

43. The pressure ventilation modes that have time triggering include:

_____

44. The pressure ventilation modes that allow for patient triggering include:

_____

45. Flow cycling is used by which pressure ventilation modes?

_____

46. Time cycling is used by which pressure ventilation modes?

_____

47. What are the advantages and disadvantages of using pressure ventilation?

_____

_____

_____

_____

48. Explain the use of low levels of PEEP for ventilator patients with COPD.

_____

_____

_____

_____

49. During pressure ventilation, how is tidal volume established?

_____

50. A patient on PC-CMV has a PIP setting of 18 cm H_2O. The V_T is measured as 400 mL. The desired V_T is 750 mL. How should the pressure be adjusted to achieve the desired V_T?

_____

_____

51. A patient on PC-CMV has a PIP setting of 14 cm H_2O. The V_T is measured as 550 mL. The desired V_T is 800 mL. How should the pressure be adjusted to achieve the desired V_T?

_____

_____

_____

_____

52. What formula can be used to estimate the level of pressure support needed for a patient?

_____

53. During VC-CMV, f = 12 b/m and V_T = 600 mL the patient's PIP was measured at 28 cm H_2O and the $P_{plateau}$ = 20 cm H_2O. The patient is now ready for VC-SIMV with pressure support. The most appropriate pressure support level to start this patient with is:

_____

54. Refer to Figure 6-2. Identify the problem on the pressure-time graph of a COPD patient receiving CPAP +5 cm H_2O with pressure support ventilation.

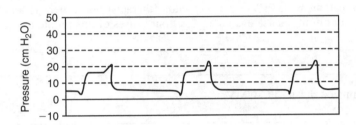

_____

55. What can be done to correct the problem identified in Question 54?

_____

56. The flow cycling percentage is set to 20% and the peak inspiratory flow is 50 L/min. At what flow rate will the ventilator cycle to exhalation?

_____

57. The flow cycling percentage is set to 40% and the peak inspiratory flow is 50 L/min. At what flow rate will the ventilator cycle to exhalation?

_____

58. Compare the answers for Questions 56 and 57. Which PS setup will provide the shortest inspiratory time? Why?

_____

_____

59. What are the three ways of establishing the initial PIP during PCV?

a. _____

b. _____

c. _____

Chapter **6** **Initial Ventilator Settings**

60. a. What are the initial setting ranges for bilevel PAP?

    b. What is the target tidal volume during bilevel PAP?

    a. _____

    b. _____

61. The ventilator mode where the breath is pressure-limited, time-cycled, and uses V_T as a feedback control is

_____.

62. How does the Servo^i establish initial pressure in the PRVC mode?

_____

_____

63. Why is it important to set an upper pressure limit during PRVC?

_____

_____

_____

64. During ventilation of a patient with PRVC the respiratory therapist notes there is an audible alarm and a digital message that says "pressure limit, please evaluate." List four causes of this problem.

_____

_____

65. Explain how P_{alv} is estimated during PC-CMV.

_____

_____

CRITICAL THINKING QUESTIONS

1. What considerations need to be made by the respiratory therapist prior to initiating mechanical ventilation?

_____

_____

_____

2. Explain why tubing compression factor is of clinical importance.

_____

_____

3. For which type of patient is volume lost from tubing compression most critical?

_____

_____

4. How do changes in compliance affect the airway pressure and exhaled tidal volume in the volume control mode compared to the pressure control mode?

_____

_____

5. What two safety systems do ventilators have to end inspiration during PSV?

_____

_____

_____

_____

CASE STUDIES

Case Study 1

A 28-year-old woman presents to the ED with complaints of general muscle weakness, dysphagia, and difficulty breathing. History of present illness reveals that she was diagnosed with infectious mononucleosis 10 days ago and has recently experienced ptosis and weakness in her legs and arms. She weighs 150 lb and is 5 foot 8 inches tall. ABG analysis on room air reveals: pH 7.30, $PaCO_2$ 50 mm Hg, PO_2 78 mm Hg, SaO_2 83%, HCO_3^- 23 mEq/L. MIP is 15 cm H_2O and VC is 13 mL/kg.

1. What is the most appropriate action at this time?

_____

2. Calculate the patient's minute ventilation using the Dubois Body Surface Chart in Figure 6-1.

_____

3. What tidal volume and respiratory rate ranges would be appropriate for this patient?

_____

Fifteen minutes later the patient's breathing is very shallow; she is unresponsive and is immediately intubated.

4. Which type of ventilation is most appropriate for this patient?

_____

5. What ventilator settings are appropriate?

_____

Case Study 2

An 8-year-old boy requires mechanical ventilation following surgical repair of his broken femur and humerus. His IBW is 80 lb. The respiratory therapist sets the ventilator to deliver 250 mL at 12 b/m with +3 cm H_2O PEEP in VC-SIMV, occludes the patient Y connector, and manually triggers a breath. The PIP reading is 68 cm H_2O.

1. Calculate the compliance factor for this circuit.

_____

The patient is then connected to the ventilator and the PIP is 27 cm H_2O.

2. Calculate the volume lost.

_____

3. Calculate the delivered V_T.

_____

4. How can the respiratory therapist compensate for this lost V_T?

_____

NBRC–STYLE QUESTIONS

1. A 6-foot-tall male patient with pulmonary fibrosis is being ventilated with VC-CMV, rate 10 b/m, V_T 600 mL, F_IO_2 50%, PEEP +10 cm H_2O. The patient's PIP is 53 cm H_2O and the $P_{plateau}$ is 47 cm H_2O. It is decided to switch the patient to PC-CMV. What set PIP will deliver 6 mL/kg IBW?
   a. 30 cm H_2O
   b. 35 cm H_2O
   c. 38 cm H_2O
   d. 43 cm H_2O

2. The most appropriate initial settings for a 5 foot 4 inches tall female postoperative patient with no lung disease would be which of the following?
   a. PC-CMV, PIP 35 cm H_2O, f 20 b/m, PEEP + 10 cm H_2O
   b. PC-SIMV, PIP 20 cm H_2O, f 6 b/m, PEEP +8 cm H_2O
   c. VC-CMV, 570 mL, f 10 b/m, PEEP +5 cm H_2O
   d. VC-CMV, 700 mL, f 14, PEEP 0

3. A patient is ready to be changed from VC-SIMV to PSV. The VC-SIMV settings were V_T 450 mL, f 4 b/m, and PEEP +5 cm H_2O. The patient's PIP is 31 cm H_2O and $P_{plateau}$ is 23 cm H_2O. The initial PSV setting for this patient should be which of the following?
   a. 5 cm H_2O
   b. 8 cm H_2O
   c. 10 cm H_2O
   d. 12 cm H_2O

4. The flow waveform that is most appropriate for a patient with high Raw is which of the following?
   a. Rectangle
   b. Descending
   c. Ascending
   d. Exponential

5. Calculate the I:E ratio when the set rate is 35 b/m and the $T_I = 1$ second.
   a. 1:1
   b. 1.4:1
   c. 1.7:1
   d. 2:1

6. What flow rate is necessary to deliver a V_T 500 mL at a rate of 15 b/m with an I:E ratio of 1:3?
   a. 30 L/min
   b. 35 L/min
   c. 40 L/min
   d. 45 L/min

7. The appropriate minute ventilation for a male with a BSA of $2.3\,m^2$ and a body temperature of $40°\,C$ is which of the following?
   a. 8.2 L/min
   b. 9.6 L/min
   c. 10.6 L/min
   d. 11.7 L/min

8. A 5 foot 1 inch tall female patient receiving PSV $6\,cmH_2O$ is showing signs of accessory muscle use and is exhaling a V_T of 220 mL at a rate of 28 b/m. The most appropriate action at this time is which of the following?
   a. Adjust the F_IO_2
   b. Increase the set flow rate
   c. Increase the PSV to $10\,cmH_2O$
   d. Adjust the flow cycling percent

9. Calculate the delivered V_T when the tubing compliance is $3.3\,cmH_2O$, the set V_T is 375 mL, and the PIP is $18\,cmH_2O$.
   a. 300 mL
   b. 316 mL
   c. 357 mL
   d. 365 mL

10. A 5 foot 7 inches tall female multiple trauma patient was being managed on VC-CMV, f 12 b/m, V_T 640 mL, PEEP $+5\,cmH_2O$, F_IO_2 60%, and a constant waveform for the past 24 hours. Currently, PIP is $45\,cmH_2O$, $P_{plateau}$ is $38\,cmH_2O$, and the patient has been diagnosed with ARDS. The respiratory therapist wants to switch the patient to PC-CMV. The initial pressure setting to target the appropriate V_T for this patient is which of the following?
    a. $10\,cm\,H_2O$
    b. $20\,cm\,H_2O$
    c. $38\,cm\,H_2O$
    d. $45\,cm\,H_2O$

7 Final Considerations in Ventilator Setup

Upon completion of this chapter, the reader will be able to do the following:

1. Recommend fractional inspired oxygen concentration F_IO_2 settings when initiating mechanical ventilation.
2. Discuss the pros and cons of using the sigh function during mechanical ventilation.
3. Compare the use of sigh with the concept of a recruitment maneuver in acute respiratory distress syndrome.
4. List the actions necessary for final ventilator setup.
5. Explain the concept of using extrinsic positive end-expiratory pressure (PEEP) in patients with airflow obstruction and air trapping who have trouble triggering a breath during mechanical ventilation.
6. Calculate the desired F_IO_2 setting given the current partial arterial pressure of oxygen (PaO_2) and F_IO_2 values.
7. List the essential capabilities of an adult intensive care unit (ICU) ventilator.
8. Provide initial ventilator settings from the guidelines for patient management for any of the following patient conditions: chronic obstructive pulmonary disease (COPD), neuromuscular disorders, acute asthma episodes, closed head injuries, ARDS, and acute cardiogenic pulmonary edema.

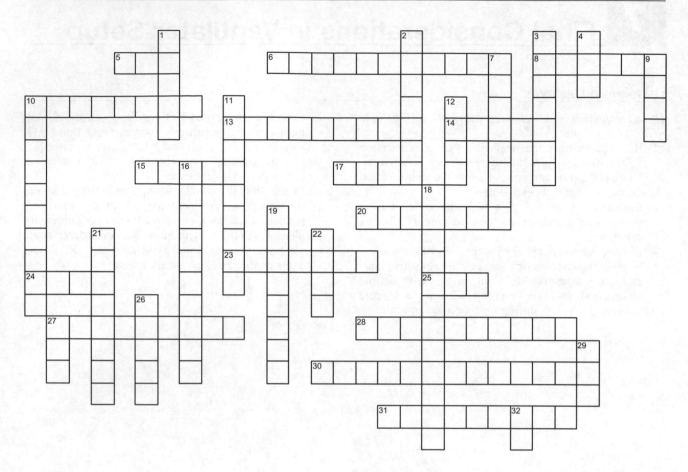

Across

5 The type of pressure measured with a closed head injury (abbreviation)
6 Pharmacologic agent that can improve myocardial oxygenation and reduce preload and afterload
8 The color of sputum in the presence of respiratory infection
10 The sound made by alveoli popping open during inspiration
13 A pharmacologic agent given to improve cardiac contractility
14 Warn of possible dangers
15 Too much air in the lungs causes this type of resonance
17 The preferred method of patient trigger that has a rapid response time
20 Type of water with which a humidifier is filled
23 The normal response to acute increases in ICP
24 A chemical administered to keep pH range acceptable (abbreviation)
25 The pressure required to maintain cerebral blood flow (abbreviation)
27 The process of adding fluids
28 Excess pressure in the lungs can cause this
30 Not in sync
31 Low amount of oxygen in the blood

Down

1 Type of alarm that warns when the patient stops breathing
2 Type of score used to evaluate a patient's neurological responses
3 Type of hyperinflation that occurs with auto-PEEP
4 The neuomuscular disease that was made famous by a ball player (abbreviation)
7 The type of humidity that is a percentage of absolute humidity compared to capacity
9 A humidifier that uses capillary action
10 Presence of this in the circuit tubing can potentially be a source of accidental lavage
11 Type of medication given to reduce vascular fluid load
12 Interface for noninvasive ventilation
16 Knowingly allowing carbon dioxide levels to rise during mechanical ventilation is known as _____ hypercapnia
18 A look-and-see type of pulmonary diagnostic procedure
19 One type of humidifier
21 Type of deficit that increases when dry gas is inhaled
22 This type of breath is used for lung recruitment
26 Type of alarm that warns when I time exceeds E time
27 An artificial nose (abbreviation)
29 The point at which inhaled air reaches 100% RH (abbreviation)
32 A neuromuscular disease with rapid onset (abbreviation)

CHAPTER REVIEW QUESTIONS

1. The clinically acceptable arterial oxygen tension range is _____.

2. Prior to elective intubation, a patient's PaO_2 was 92 mm Hg with a nasal cannula running at 2 L/min. What F_IO_2 should be set on the ventilator?

   _____

3. Calculate the estimated F_IO_2 using the following information: known F_IO_2 50%, known PaO_2 60 mm Hg, desired PaO_2 90 mm Hg.

   _____

   _____

   _____

4. What F_IO_2 should be set on the ventilator for a post-cardiac arrest patient?

   _____

5. What is the acceptable goal for SpO_2?

   _____

6. How long after placement on a ventilator should a blood gas be drawn on a patient?

   _____

7. Use of high concentrations of oxygen can cause what three problems?

   a. _____

   b. _____

   c. _____

8. Why does flow triggering have a faster response time than pressure triggering?

   _____

   _____

9. How does auto-PEEP interfere with pressure triggering?

   _____

   _____

   _____

10. The point in the tracheobronchial tree at which inhaled gas contains 44 mg/L of water, has reached 100% relative humidity, and is 37° C is called the

    _____ and is located at the level of the

    _____.

11. The absolute humidity of a ventilator's humidification system needs to be _____

    at temperatures between _____ and

    _____.

12. What are two advantages of a closed humidification system?

    a. _____

    b. _____

13. What causes excessive rain-out (condensation) in a ventilator circuit?

    _____

    _____

    _____

    _____

14. How much water can a Heat Moisture Exchanger (HME) provide during tidal volumes of 500 to 1,000 mL?

    _____

15. How much water can a Hygroscopic HME provide during tidal volumes of 500 to 1,000 mL?

    _____

16. What happens to an HME when moisture and secretions accumulate in it?

    _____

    _____

17. What should be done with the HME during an aerosol treatment using a small volume nebulizer? How can this be avoided?

    _____

    _____

18. An MDI with a spacer should be placed where in a ventilator circuit? What should be done with the HME?

_____

_____

_____

19. List at least four contraindications for the use of HMEs.

a. _____

b. _____

c. _____

d. _____

20. What are the three levels of alarms and their descriptions?

_____

_____

For Questions 21–36, identify the alarm situations with the appropriate alarm level: **select 1, 2, or 3**.

21. _____ Heater/humidifier malfunction

22. _____ Timing failure

23. _____ Autocycling

24. _____ Auto-PEEP

25. _____ Excessive gas delivery to patient

26. _____ Inappropriate PEEP/CPAP

27. _____ Exhalation valve failure

28. _____ I:E ratio inappropriate

29. _____ Electrical power failure

30. _____ Changes in lung characteristics

31. _____ Circuit leak

32. _____ No gas delivery to patient

33. _____ Electrical power failure

34. _____ Circuit partially obstructed

35. _____ Inappropriate oxygen level

36. _____ Changes in ventilatory drive

37. Following the application of a VC-CMV with $8\,cm\,H_2O$ PEEP to a patient, the respiratory therapist notices that the average PIP is $30\,cm\,H_2O$. The low-pressure, high-pressure, and low PEEP/CPAP alarms should be set at what values?

_____

38. The maximum value at which the apnea alarm should be set with any ventilator is how many seconds?

_____

39. Lung recruitment strategies and sigh maneuvers are similar in what way?

_____

_____

40. List four circumstances for which sighs or deep breaths are appropriate?

a. _____

b. _____

c. _____

d. _____

41. List the necessary considerations (10) for preparation of final ventilator setup.

a. _____

b. _____

c. _____

d. _____

e. _____

f. _____

g. _____

h. _____

i. _____

j. _____

42. List the essential capabilities of an adult ventilator.

Modes: _____

Tidal volume range: _____

Respiratory rate range: _____

Pressure range: _____

PEEP/CPAP range: _____

Flow rate range: _____

Flow waveforms: _____

F_1O_2: _____

Diagnostic measurements: _____

Alarms: _____

43. What lung characteristics do patients with COPD exhibit?

_____

44. What is the primary reason for mechanical ventilatory support for patients with COPD?

_____

45. List at least five causes of increased morbidity for COPD patients receiving ventilatory support.

a. _____

b. _____

c. _____

d. _____

e. _____

46. The mode of choice for a patient with COPD, if possible, is _____.

47. The intubation route of choice for a patient with COPD is _____.

48. Complete the following chart summarizing the ventilator guidelines for COPD patients:

Parameter	Preferred Setting or Range
Tidal volume	_____
Rate	_____
Inspiratory time	_____
Flow rate	_____
Flow waveform	_____
PEEP	_____
F_1O_2	_____

49. List at least five neuromuscular disorders that may require ventilatory support.

a. _____

b. _____

c. _____

d. _____

e. _____

50. What are the main reasons why patients with these neuromuscular disorders require ventilatory support?

_____

_____

51. Complete the following chart summarizing the ventilator guidelines for patients with neuromuscular disorders:

Parameter	Preferred Setting or Range
Tidal volume	_____
Rate	_____
Inspiratory time	_____
Flow rate	_____
Flow waveform	_____
PEEP	_____
F_1O_2	_____

52. Define *pulsus paradoxus*.

_____

_____

_____

53. What are the two main concerns that a respiratory therapist must be aware of during the mechanical ventilation of a patient with acute asthma?

a. _____

b. _____

54. During ventilation of a patient with asthma, plateau pressure should be kept at _____.

55. The pharmacological agents that may be used to keep pH greater than 7.20 while using permissive hypercapnia are _____ and

_____.

56. Complete the following chart summarizing the ventilator guidelines for patients with acute severe asthma:

Parameter	Preferred Setting or Range
Tidal volume	_____
Rate	_____
Inspiratory time	_____
Flow rate	_____
Flow waveform	_____
PEEP	_____
F_1O_2	_____

57. Diagnostic percussion during an asthma episode will reveal _____.

58. What are the common causes of increased intracranial pressures?

_____

_____

_____

_____

59. The equation for cerebral perfusion pressure is

_____

60. What are the normal values for the components of this formula?

_____

_____

61. What CPP indicates poor cerebral perfusion?

_____

_____

62. When and how should iatrogenic hyperventilation be used?

_____

_____

63. Complete the following chart summarizing the ventilator guidelines for patients with closed head injury:

Parameter	Preferred Setting or Range
Tidal volume	_____
Rate	_____
Inspiratory time	_____
Flow rate	_____
Flow waveform	_____
PEEP	_____
F_1O_2	_____

64. What is the open lung approach to ventilating patients with ARDS?

_____

_____

_____

65. Complete the following chart summarizing the ventilator guidelines for patients with ARDS:

Parameter	Preferred Setting or Range
Tidal volume	_____
Rate	_____
Inspiratory time	_____
Flow rate	_____
Flow waveform	_____
PEEP	_____
F_1O_2	_____

66. In the management of ARDS, what are the acceptable end points for arterial blood gases?

_____

_____

_____

67. List at least seven examples of precipitating conditions associated with the development of ARDS.

a. _____

b. _____

c. _____

d. _____

e. _____

f. _____

g. _____

68. How is refractory hypoxemia identified?

_____

_____

_____

69. How does ARDS present on chest x-ray?

_____

_____

_____

70. A patient with ARDS will have a total lung compliance of less than _____ cm H_2O.

71. The amount of pulmonary shunt that is indicative of

    ARDS is _____.

72. The pulmonary capillary wedge pressure values that are typically found in patients with ARDS are

    _____.

73. Five common causes of acute pulmonary edema include:

    a. _____

    b. _____

    c. _____

    d. _____

    e. _____

74. Complete the following chart summarizing the ventilator guidelines for patients with CHF:

Parameter	Preferred Setting or Range
Tidal volume	_____
Rate	_____
Inspiratory time	_____
Flow rate	_____
Flow waveform	_____
PEEP	_____
F_IO_2	_____

75. Patients with congestive heart failure and mild to moderate hypoxemia can be successfully managed without intubation using what two modalities?

    _____

    _____

    _____

CRITICAL THINKING QUESTIONS

1. Discuss the pros and cons for using sighs with mechanical ventilation.

    _____

    _____

    _____

    _____

    _____

2. Explain the progression of an asthma episode from arrival at the ED to being intubated and mechanically ventilated.

    _____

    _____

    _____

    _____

    _____

    _____

    _____

3. Discuss why the use of PSV may not be appropriate for patients with COPD.

    _____

    _____

    _____

    _____

    _____

    _____

    _____

4. Why does the exhalation valve not have to close at the beginning of a flow-triggered breath?

    _____

    _____

    _____

5. Why is it important for expiratory time to be maximized when ventilating a patient with increased airway resistance, such as with asthma or COPD?

    _____

    _____

    _____

Chapter **7** **Final Considerations in Ventilator Setup**

Case Study 1

A 62-year-old male weighing 256 lbs is 73 inches tall. The patient has a history of congestive heart failure and is placed on a non-rebreathing mask. Physical assessment reveals a patient who is alert and oriented, but anxious and diaphoretic. Pulse 142 beats/min and thready, blood pressure 105/68, temperature 98.6° F, respiratory rate 26 shallow and labored. Breath sounds reveal bilateral inspiratory coarse crackles. The ABG on the non-rebreathing mask is pH 7.24, $PaCO_2$ 51 mm Hg, PaO_2 42 mm Hg, and HCO_3^- 23 mEq/L. The patient's electrocardiogram shows a widened QRS complex with occasional premature ventricular contractions.

1. What respiratory care intervention is indicated at this time?

   _____

   _____

2. If this patient was to be intubated and placed on mechanical ventilation, what mode, tidal volume, and rate would be appropriate?

   _____

   _____

Case Study 2

A motor vehicle accident victim arrives at the hospital via ambulance. This 37-year-old patient has sustained a closed-head injury. Physical assessment reveals pulse 145 beats/min, respiratory rate 32 breaths/min, and blood pressure 155/97. Her neck veins are distended; she is diaphoretic and anxious. She is 68 inches tall and weighs 175 lbs. The patient has no history of cardiac or respiratory disease. The patient has an oral airway in place and has a weak gag reflex. On 60% oxygen, the arterial blood gases are: pH 7.22, $PaCO_2$ 64 mm Hg, PaO_2 78 mm Hg, SaO_2 92%, and HCO_3^- 25 mEq/L

1. What type of respiratory failure appears to be present in this patient?

   _____

   _____

2. What acid-base imbalance is present?

   _____

3. What type of mechanical ventilatory support should benefit this patient?

   _____

4. What are the appropriate parameters for this patient, including minute ventilation, tidal volume, inspiratory time, flow rate, and PEEP?

   _____

   _____

   _____

Case Study 3

A 40-year-old female, height 66 inches, and weight 156 lbs is admitted to the ED. She is alert, very anxious, unable to complete a sentence without stopping to take a breath, and is sitting in a tripod position. Her heart rate is 136 beats/min and regular, respirations 30/min and very labored with accessory muscle use. Blood pressure is 168/84 and temperature is 37.2° C. Breath sounds are decreased bilaterally with expiratory wheezes. She has a weak, nonproductive cough. The patient has been receiving continuous aerosol albuterol and has a Solu-Medrol IV. The patient's best peak flow following bronchodilator therapy is 65 L/min. ABG results while on nasal cannula 6 L/min show pH 7.34, $PaCO_2$ 42 mm Hg, PaO_2 48 mm Hg, SaO_2 79%, and HCO_3^- 22 mEq/L.

1. How should this blood gas be interpreted?

   _____

   _____

   _____

2. Does the situation warrant intubation and mechanical ventilation? Why or why not?

   _____

   _____

   _____

3. What type of mechanical ventilatory support should benefit this patient?

   _____

   _____

   _____

4. If PC-CMV is used for this patient, what are the appropriate settings (including PIP setting, resulting tidal volume, respiratory rate, inspiratory time, waveform, and PEEP)?

   _____

   _____

   _____

Case Study 4

A 64-year-old, 197-lb, 6-foot 1-inch male patient was admitted three days ago for a COPD exacerbation. He is currently receiving supplemental oxygen via nasal cannula at 3 L/min; albuterol and ipratropium every 4 hours; and is receiving an intravenous corticosteroid and antibiotic. He has bilaterally diminished breath sounds with rhonchi in both bases. He has a weak nonproductive cough. A chest x-ray from this morning shows bibasilar infiltrates. The current ABG results reveal: pH 7.32, $PaCO_2$ 57 mm Hg, PaO_2 54 mm Hg, SaO_2 85%, and HCO_3^- 28 mEq/L.

1. How should this blood gas be interpreted?

_____

2. Does the situation warrant intubation and mechanical ventilation? Why or why not?

_____

_____

_____

3. If intubation is required what mode and parameters should be used for this patient?

_____

_____

_____

NBRC–STYLE QUESTIONS

1. Which of the following is (are) true concerning the use of permissive hypercapnia in the management of ARDS?
   1. Bicarbonate may be administered to keep pH >7.20
   2. $PaCO_2$ should go no higher than 60 mm Hg
   3. The pH may be allowed to drop as low as 7.10
   4. The $PaCO_2$ is permitted to rise rapidly to the acceptable level
   a. 1 and 3 only
   b. 2 and 4 only
   c. 1 and 4 only
   d. 2 and 3 only

2. A mechanically ventilated patient has been using an HME for humidification for the past 72 hours. On rounds the respiratory therapist notices a steady increase in PIP over the past two days. The respiratory therapist suctions the patient to assess the patient's secretions. The secretions are very thick and tenacious. The most appropriate action at this time is which of the following?
   a. Suction the patient more often.
   b. Add a passover humidifier to the system.
   c. Switch to a heated wick-type humidifier.
   d. Use normal saline to lavage before suctioning.

3. A 75-year-old female, admitted through the ED earlier today, is increasingly distressed and unable to breathe comfortably except in the upright position. She has a history of coronary artery disease, and on admission was complaining of chest pain. She is becoming increasingly short of breath and appears cyanotic. Vital signs reveal: pulse 142 beats/min, blood pressure 150/92, respiratory rate 30 and labored. The ABG on nasal cannula 3 L/min is pH 7.18, $PaCO_2$ 81 mm Hg, PaO_2 35 mm Hg, SaO_2 79%, and HCO_3^- 29 mEq/L. The respiratory therapist should recommend which of the following?
   a. Nasal mask CPAP at 10 cm H_2O
   b. Non-rebreathing mask with 15 L/min oxygen
   c. Bilevel PAP: IPAP 15 cm H_2O and EPAP 5 cm H_2O
   d. Intubation and mechanical ventilation with PC-CMV

4. Appropriate ventilatory parameters for an otherwise healthy 185-lb, 6-foot 1-inch, 26-year-old male patient who was brought to the ED because of a drug overdose include which of the following?
   a. VC-CMV, tidal volume 1.0L, set rate 8 breaths/min
   b. VC-SIMV, tidal volume 600 mL, set rate 6 breaths/min
   c. PC-CMV, set pressure 25 cm H_2O, inspiratory time 1.5 sec
   d. Pressure support ventilation of 15 cm H_2O with CPAP 5 cm H_2O

5. Prior to intubation a patient's PaO_2 was 78 mm Hg while receiving an F_IO_2 of 60%. What F_IO_2 setting on the ventilator will bring the PaO_2 up to 90 mm Hg? (Assume that this patient's cardiopulmonary status and respiratory quotient are constant.)
   a. 70%
   b. 75%
   c. 80%
   d. 85%

6. A patient has just been intubated in the ED. The patient is a 64-year-old obese male patient with a suspected drug overdose. The patient is 6 feet tall and weighs 435 lbs. The most appropriate tidal volume to ventilate this patient is which of the following?
   a. 380 mL
   b. 640 mL
   c. 810 mL
   d. 975 mL

7. Which of the following ventilatory parameters is appropriate when mechanically ventilating a patient with COPD?
   a. Use a rectangle flow waveform.
   b. Set tidal volume between 10 and 15 mL/kg.
   c. Use peak inspiratory flow rates >60 L/min.
   d. Institute PEEP in the range of 5 to 10 cm H_2O.

63

8. A patient with ARDS has been changed from VC-CMV to PC-CMV. When this change was made, there was an increase in mean airway pressure. Which of the following statements is true concerning elevated mean airway pressures?
   a. The mean airway pressure increases with longer expiratory times.
   b. An increased mean airway pressure may result in improved oxygenation.
   c. Elevated mean airway pressures decrease the risk of barotraumas.
   d. High mean airway pressures increase the risk of cardiovascular side effects.

9. A 5 feet 4 inches tall, 125 lb female patient who has just been intubated due to a severe asthma episode would be ventilated most appropriately with which of the following ventilator parameters?
   a. PSV 20 cm H_2O with CPAP 10 cm H_2O
   b. PC-CMV, 8 breaths/min, PIP 25 cm H_2O, T_I 0.75 sec, descending waveform
   c. VC-SIMV, 12 breaths/min, V_T 800 mL, flow 50 L/min, rectangle waveform
   d. VC-CMV, 10 breaths/min, V_T 570 mL, flow 35 L/min, descending waveform

10. HMEs may not be appropriate for use with infants, children, and small adults due to which of the following?
    a. Presence of mechanical dead space in the HMEs
    b. Increased rate of ET occlusion with these patients
    c. Patients' inability to overcome resistance across the HME
    d. HMEs' inability to provide adequate humidity for these patients

8 | Initial Patient Assessment

LEARNING OBJECTIVES

Upon completion of this chapter, the reader will be able to do the following:

1. Understand the importance of performing an operational verification procedure.
2. State the recommended times when an oxygen analyzer is used to measure the fractional inspired oxygen concentration (F_IO_2) during mechanical ventilation.
3. Identify various pathophysiologic conditions that alter a patient's transairway pressure, peak pressure, and plateau pressure.
4. Use pressure-time and flow-time curves obtained during pressure-controlled continuous mandatory ventilation to determine the plateau pressure.
5. Identify a system leak from a volume-time curve.
6. Use physical examination and radiographic data to determine whether pneumonia, acute respiratory distress syndrome (ARDS), flail chest, pneumothorax, asthma, pleural effusion, or emphysema is present.
7. Determine whether a lung compliance problem or an airway resistance problem is present using

the ventilator flow sheet and time, volume, peak inspiratory pressure (PIP), and plateau pressure data.
8. Evaluate a static pressure–volume curve for static compliance and dynamic compliance to determine changes in compliance or resistance.
9. Estimate a patient's alveolar ventilation based on ideal body weight, tidal volume, and respiratory rate.
10. Detect a cuff leak by listening to breath sounds.
11. Recognize inappropriate endotracheal tube cuff pressures and an inappropriate tube size and recommend measures to correct these problems.
12. Evaluate flow sheet information about a patient on pressure control ventilation and recommend methods for determining whether compliance and airway resistance have changed.
13. Explain the technique for measuring endotracheal tube cuff pressure using a manometer, syringe, and three-way stopcock.
14. Describe two methods that can be used to remedy a cut pilot tube (pilot balloon line) without changing the endotracheal tube.

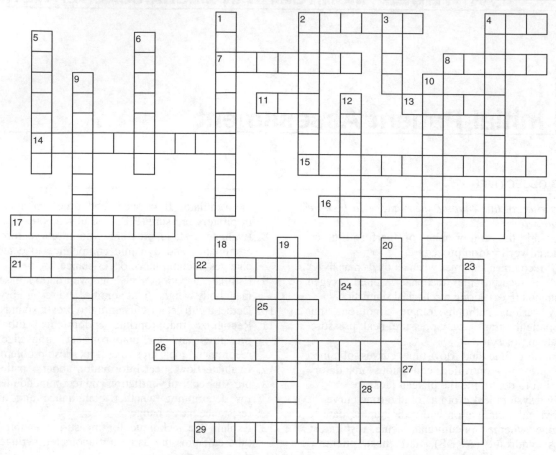

Across

2 A place to measure temperature
4 Something in the ventilator circuit that adds dead space (abbreviation)
7 A cause of abdominal distention due to fluid
8 The _____ inflection point indicates a time at which large numbers of alveoli are becoming over-inflated
11 A test to check that a ventilator is working properly (abbreviation)
13 An endotracheal tube has a _____ balloon
14 A common place for leaks
15 It puts air in the pleural space and reduces lung compliance
16 The setting that allows patient triggering
17 Cell death
21 The _____ inflection point indicates the pressure at which large numbers of alveoli are being recruited
22 Type of compliance measured at no flow
24 Type of compliance that is measured during gas movement
25 A pressure that can be measured continuously by a flow-directed catheter (abbreviation)
26 What's left in the tubing is called _____ volume
27 Another name for base flow is _____ flow
29 The form on which the patient-ventilator check is written (two words)

Down

1 Type of pressure that is important to tissue oxygenation and affects both lung volumes and cardiac output (two words)
2 Dynamic hyperinflation (two words)
3 When exhaled tidal volume is less than set tidal volume there is a _____
4 A condition of low body temperature
5 A breath sound that indicates the possible need for suctioning
6 A type of recoil
9 It puts fluid in the alveoli and reduces lung compliance (two words)
10 A place where the central venous pressure catheter dwells (two words)
12 A breath sound that indicates the possible need for bronchodilator therapy
18 The amount of pressure needed to overcome airway resistance (abbreviation)
19 Heart rate, respiratory rate, and blood pressure are all part of this (two words)
20 Tidal volume times frequency equals _____ ventilation
23 The secondary respiratory muscles
28 Method for ensuring no leaks around an endotracheal tube (abbreviation)

CHAPTER REVIEW QUESTIONS

1. List some of the observations of a mechanically ventilated patient that can help determine the patient's physiological statue.

   _____

   _____

   _____

   _____

2. Documentation of patient information and ventilator settings should be made on the _____.

3. Before a ventilator can be used on a patient, a therapist must perform what type of procedure?

   _____

4. In addition to regularly timed checks, list 6 instances when patient-ventilator system checks should be performed:

   a. _____

   b. _____

   c. _____

   d. _____

   e. _____

   f. _____

5. How often should the F_IO_2 be measured for an adult and how often for an infant? _____

6. How long should a respiratory therapist wait after the initiation of mechanical ventilation to draw an ABG sample?

   _____

7. The appropriate range for pressure trigger setting (sensitivity setting) is:

   _____

8. The appropriate range for flow triggering setting (sensitivity setting) is:

   _____

9. a. How does auto-PEEP make trigger the ventilator more difficult for a patient?

   b. How can triggering the ventilator be made easier without causing autotriggering?

   a. _____

   b. _____

10. List what strategies may be used to eliminate or reduce auto-PEEP.

    _____

    _____

    _____

11. Calculate how much volume is lost to the patient's ventilator circuit when the C_T is 3.27 mL/cm H$_2$O and the PIP is 48 cm H$_2$O.

    _____

    _____

12. What effect would an HME attached to the endotracheal tube have on alveolar ventilation?

    _____

    _____

13. Calculate the alveolar minute ventilation if the set V_T is 775 mL, ideal body weight is 160 lbs, and added V_D is 85 mL.

    _____

    _____

14. List three factors which determine alveolar ventilation.

    a. _____

    b. _____

    c. _____

15. An increase in PIP may be due to _____ in compliance or _____ in airway resistance.

16. What control must be used to measure plateau pressure?

    _____

17. Under what circumstance could an inaccurate plateau pressure measurement be obtained?

    _____

    _____

18. Dynamic compliance is calculated using what pressure measurement?

    _____

19. Static compliance is calculated using what pressure measurement?

    _____

20. Define *transairway pressure* and write the formula.

_____

_____

21. What does an increase in the difference between PIP and $P_{plateau}$ indicate?

_____

_____

22. What are the most common causes for increased airway resistance?

_____

_____

_____

23. What is the significance of monitoring mean airway pressure?

_____

_____

24. The high pressure limit alarm is usually set at about _____ cm H_2O above the measured PIP, and when activated it will _____ .

25. List the most common causes that activate the high pressure limit alarm.

_____

_____

_____

26. The low pressure alarm is usually set at _____ cm H_2O below the measured PIP, and when activated usually indicates _____ .

27. List the common causes that activate the low pressure alarm.

_____

_____

_____

28. If the leak is not obvious, the patient must be _____ while the leak is checked.

29. What two methods can the respiratory therapist use to determine whether a leak is present?

a. _____

b. _____

30. If a leak is present, what steps should be taken to find the source?

_____

_____

_____

_____

_____

31. What effect would a leak have during pressure support ventilation?

_____

32. List the factors that can affect a ventilated patient's heart rate.

_____

_____

_____

33. List the factors that can cause hyperthermia.

_____

_____

_____

34. List the factors that can cause hypothermia.

_____

_____

_____

35. The central venous pressure (CVP) directly reflects what pressures?

_____

_____

36. At what point during a ventilator breath should the CVP measurement be taken?

_____

37. What type of patient would benefit from the monitoring of pulmonary artery pressure?

_____

_____

38. How often should a physical examination of a ventilated patient be performed?

_____

39. What should be included in the physical examination?

_____

40. What effect does abdominal distention have on ventilation?

_____

41. Endotracheal or tracheostomy cuff pressure should not exceed what range?

_____

42. In what type of patient could a cuff pressure of 25 mm Hg (24 cm H_2O) cause tracheal damage?

_____

43. List the five-step protocol designed to minimize the risk of tracheal necrosis associated with cuff overinflation.

   a. _____

   b. _____

   c. _____

   d. _____

   e. _____

44. List two situations when a higher than acceptable cuff pressure may be required to maintain a minimal occlusion?

   a. _____

   b. _____

45. If it is determined that the source of a leak is either the pilot balloon or valve, the cuff can be inflated, and a _____ attached to the pilot balloon and turned to the _____ position. If the pilot balloon is still leaking, the problem can be temporarily solved by placing a _____ on the pilot line.

46. Describe the procedure for maintaining cuff pressure if the pilot balloon is accidentally cut.

_____

_____

47. What is the rationale for repositioning an endotracheal tube in the patient's mouth every 8 to 12 hours?

_____

_____

48. List the possible causes for a decrease in static compliance.

_____

_____

49. The normal value for static compliance is

_____.

50. During pressure ventilation, if the set inspiratory pressure remains constant, what effect would a decreased static compliance have on tidal volume?

_____

51. The formula for static compliance is

_____.

52. C_D decreases whenever C_S _____ or

   Raw _____.

53. The formula to calculate dynamic compliance is

_____.

54. During volume ventilation what effect would a decrease in C_D have on PIP and the delivered tidal volume?

_____

_____

_____

55. Calculate the C_S when the V_T is 740 mL, $P_{plateau}$ is 44 cm H_2O, and the end-expiratory pressure is +8 cm H_2O.

_____

_____

56. Calculate the Raw when the PIP is 58 cm H_2O, $P_{plateau}$ is 51 cm H_2O, and the flow is 0.5 L/sec.

_____

_____

57. Calculate airway resistance for a ventilated patient with the following: PIP 48 cm H_2O, $P_{plateau}$ 30 cm H_2O, and a set flow rate of 40 L/min.

_____

_____

Chapter **8** **Initial Patient Assessment**

58. Identify the problem in Figure 8-1.

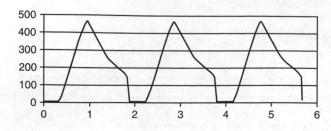

59. What is the plateau pressure in Figure 8-2?

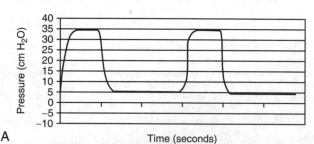

A

Time (seconds)

B

Time (seconds)

60. Calculate the static compliance for the information in Figure 8-2 using the returned tidal volume of 450 mL.

CRITICAL THINKING QUESTIONS

1. During a ventilator check the respiratory therapist notices the patient making inspiratory efforts (patient is using accessory muscles), but the ventilator is not triggering. What could be causing the problem? What steps could be taken to correct it?

2. A 250-pound adult male has a 6.5-mm (inner diameter) endotracheal tube in place and is being mechanically ventilated. Cuff pressures of 40 cm H_2O are required to maintain an adequate seal. What recommendations should be made to correct this problem?

3. A patient with ARDS is being maintained on PCV, with a set inspiratory pressure of 30 cm H_2O. According to the ventilator flow sheet, measured tidal volumes for the last 3 days have ranged between 400 and 450 mL. During the first ventilator-patient check of the day, the respiratory therapist notes that the measured tidal volume is now 550 mL, without any change in set parameters. What would cause the tidal volume to increase?

4. When the PIP is 43 cm H_2O and the plateau pressure is 18 cm H_2O, how much pressure is required to overcome the resistance of the airways?

CASE STUDIES

Case Study 1

A respiratory therapist is called to a code in the ICU. After the patient is stabilized, the physician writes the following order for mechanical ventilation: Volume control, V_T 700 mL, *f* 12, F_1O_2 100%, PEEP +5 cm H_2O. The therapist observes that the PIP is 42 cm H_2O.

1. At what levels should the high- and low-pressure alarms be set?

2. At what level should the low V_T alarm be set?

Chapter **8** **Initial Patient Assessment**

3. What would the therapist need to do to obtain a plateau pressure?

_____

4. What could the therapist conclude if the plateau pressure equals $38\,cm\,H_2O$?

_____

_____

_____

Case Study 2

An obtunded patient in the ICU has been receiving VC-CMV for the past 3 days. Today the patient appears to be awakening. The high pressure, low minute volume, and low tidal volume alarms are activating frequently, and the patient appears to be agitated and confused.

1. Indicate possible causes for the high pressure alarm activating.

_____

_____

2. If there are no leaks in the system, why are the low minute volume and low tidal volume alarms being activated?

_____

_____

3. What could be the possible underlying cause? What recommendations would you make to resolve the problem?

_____

_____

Case Study 3

A 38-year-old female patient was admitted through the ED 24 hours ago following a motor vehicle accident. She was intubated in the field due to respiratory arrest secondary to blunt chest trauma. The patient sustained four fractured ribs. The patient is currently on VC-CMV, f 15 b/min, V_T 440 mL, F_IO_2 80%, $PEEP_E$ $8\,cm\,H_2O$. The following values were obtained on those ventilator settings:

Time	PIP (cm H$_2$O)	P$_{plateau}$ (cm H$_2$O)	Exhaled V$_T$ (mL)
0800	35	30	440
1000	39	34	440
1100	45	39	440
1130	50	44	440

1. What is the P_{ta} for each patient-ventilator system check?

_____

2. What is the source of the increase in the PIP over the course of the 3.5 hours?

_____

_____

3. What are some of the most likely causes of this problem?

_____

_____

4. How would you assess the patient to determine the appropriate treatment?

_____

_____

_____

Case Study 4

A 56-year-old male patient with a history of COPD was admitted yesterday with a diagnosis of pneumonia. During the night he was intubated due to respiratory arrest. The patient is currently receiving VC-CMV, f 12 b/min, V_T 525 mL, F_IO_2 40%, $PEEP_E$ $3\,cm\,H_2O$. The following values were obtained on those ventilator settings:

Time	PIP (cm H$_2$O)	P$_{plateau}$ (cm H$_2$O)	Exhaled V$_T$ (mL)
0630	36	23	525
0835	39	22	523
1030	41	23	525
1230	46	19	524

1. What is the P_{ta} for each patient-ventilator system check?

_____

2. What is the source of the increase in PIP over the course of the 6 hours?

_____

_____

3. What are some of the most likely causes of this problem?

_____

_____

4. How would you assess and treat this patient?

_____

_____

_____

NBRC-STYLE QUESTIONS

1. An increase in the peak inspiratory flow rate would increase which of the following?
   a. Tidal volume
   b. Total cycle time
   c. Expiratory time
   d. Inspiratory time

2. A patient receiving volume-cycled mechanical ventilation has a decrease in static compliance. Which of the following would most likely occur?
   a. An increase in tidal volume
   b. A decrease in minute ventilation
   c. An increase in PIP
   d. An increased I:E ratio

3. While monitoring endotracheal cuff pressures during a ventilator check, the therapist maintains a reading of $44\,cm\,H_2O$. What should the therapist do next?
   a. Get a syringe and add air to the cuff.
   b. Insert a smaller diameter endotracheal tube.
   c. No changes need to be made; the cuff pressure is acceptable.
   d. Release air from the cuff until minimal occluding volume is achieved.

4. Which of the following can cause a mechanically ventilated patient's peak inspiratory pressure to increase from 20 to $40\,cm\,H_2O$ while the static compliance remains relatively unchanged?
   a. Removed mucous plugs
   b. Increased airway resistance
   c. Tension pneumothorax
   d. Decreased elastance

5. An increase in PIP and plateau pressure with a stable transairway pressure may be caused by which of the following?
   a. Acute respiratory distress syndrome
   b. Acute asthma exacerbation
   c. Retained secretions in the airways
   d. Too small an endotracheal tube

6. When responding to a ventilator alarm, the respiratory therapist sees that the low-pressure alarm is activated. She hears an audible leak, and notices that the exhaled volume is $200\,mL$ below the set tidal volume. The measured cuff pressure is $15\,mm\,Hg$. What action should be taken next?
   a. Replace the endotracheal tube with a larger size.
   b. Increase the patient's V_T to compensate for the leak.

   c. Instill enough volume into the cuff to maintain a pressure of $30\,cm\,H_2O$.
   d. While auscultating the larynx, instill enough air into the cuff until a slight leak is heard on inspiration.

7. Why is end-expiratory pressure subtracted from plateau pressure when calculating C_s?
   a. To compensate for a loss in volume due to a leak
   b. To determine auto-PEEP
   c. To determine the actual pressure change
   d. To calculate the actual PEEP level

8. Which of the following may cause an increase in heart rate?
   1. Hypoxemia
   2. Hypothermia
   3. Anxiety
   4. Pain
   a. 1 only
   b. 1 and 3 only
   c. 1, 2, and 3 only
   d. 1, 3, and 4 only

9. Which of the following physical findings would you expect when assessing an asthmatic patient?
   1. Late inspiratory crackles
   2. Hyperresonant percussion note
   3. Accessory muscle use
   4. Tracheal shift
   a. 1 only
   b. 1 and 3
   c. 2 and 3
   d. 2, 3, and 4

10. Evaluate the following data from the patient's flow sheet:

Time	Set V_T	PIP (cm H_2O)	$P_{plateau}$ (cm H_2O)
4:00	700 mL	38	32
5:00	700 mL	41	34
6:00	700 mL	47	32

Which of the following statements is true?
   a. C_L is improving.
   b. There is no change in C_L.
   c. Raw is improving.
   d. There is an increase in Raw.

9 Ventilator Graphics

Upon completion of this chapter, the reader will be able to do the following:

1. Identify ventilator variables (e.g., the target variable and trigger variable) and ventilator parameters and their values (e.g., peak inspiratory pressure and plateau pressure) using pressure, flow, and volume scalars generated using various modes of mechanical ventilation.

2. Identify ventilator variables and ventilator parameters and their values from flow-volume and pressure-volume loops.

3. Use ventilator scalars and loops to identify changes in lung compliance and airway resistance, inappropriate sensitivity settings, inadequate inspiratory flow, auto-PEEP, leaks in the ventilator circuit, active exhalation during pressure support ventilation, and an inspiratory pressure overshoot during pressure-support ventilation.

4. Calculate airway resistance and lung compliance using values derived from scalars and loops generated during mechanical ventilation.

5. Describe the changes that occur in scalars and loops during volume-targeted and pressure-targeted ventilation when airway resistance increases and lung compliance decreases.

6. Given a compliance value obtained during pressure-controlled ventilation, determine tidal volume delivery and recommend ways to adjust the set pressure to gain a desired tidal volume.

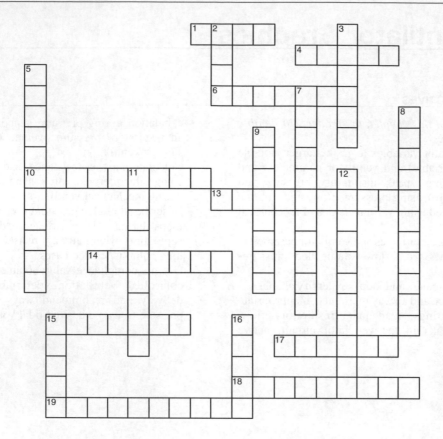

Across

1 Volume per unit of time
4 This control adjusts the rate at which the flow valve opens
6 Pressure reading when inspiration is held
10 Easy to inflate
13 Lagging of two associated phenomena
14 Begins inspiration
15 Another name for a graph
17 One variable plotted against time
18 When not asynchronous
19 Opposition to ventilation

Down

2 Two variables, other than time, plotted against each other.
3 Flow multiplied by inspiratory time
5 When patient and ventilator are not working together
7 Rapid rise or decay on a graph
8 Name of pressure gradient required to overcome airway resistance
9 Type of flow that creates a waveform parallel to the x axis
11 Type of PEEP caused by air trapping
12 A square wave is also known as _____
15 Adjusting the rise of pressure or flow to the patient
16 This is necessary to measure plateau pressure

1. Identify the scalar shapes in Figure 9-1.

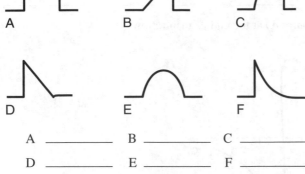

A _____ B _____ C _____

D _____ E _____ F _____

2. What is the difference between a scalar and a loop?

_____

3. What is the mathematical relationship between volume, flow, and inspiratory time?

_____

4. What two factors determine the flow of gas into the lungs?

   a. _____

   b. _____

5. As lung compliance increases, the pressure required to deliver the volume to the patient _____. When lung compliance decreases, the pressure required to deliver the volume to the patient _____.

6. The pressure at the mouth (P_{awo}) is equal to the sum of what two pressures?

_____

7. When does the flow-time curve run parallel to the x axis?

_____

8. Calculate the T_I in seconds when the volume is 600 mL and the flow rate is 60 L/min.

_____

9. Calculate P_{alv} when the delivered volume is 800 mL and static compliance is 25 mL/cm H_2O.

_____

10. Identify the labeled parts of the flow-time scalar in Figure 9-2.

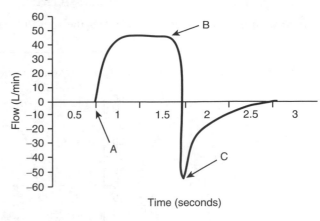

A _____

B _____

C _____

For Questions 11 through 14, refer to the flow waveform in Figure 9-3.

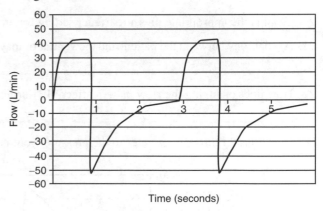

11. What type of flow waveform is shown in the figure?

_____

12. What is the peak inspiratory flow rate?

_____

13. What is the peak expiratory flow rate?

_____

14. What is the approximate inspiratory time? _____

_____

15. What is the expiratory time? _____

16. _____ prevents the flow curve from returning to zero at the end of exhalation.

17. What would invalidate an auto-PEEP measurement?

_____

18. At what point in the breath cycle does the auto-PEEP measurement occur?

_____

19. In Figure 9-4, what is the reason for the increase in flow (*point A*) at the end of inspiration?

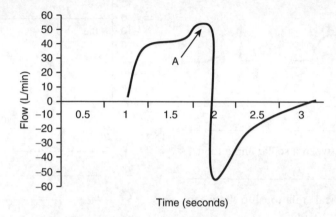

_____

20. What is the appropriate pressure trigger setting for an adult patient? _____

21. Asynchrony between the patient and the ventilator may be caused by inappropriate settings of which two parameters?

_____

22. How does changing the flow pattern affect PIP during volume ventilation?

_____

For Questions 23 through 29, refer to the pressure, volume, and flow curves for VC-CMV in the graphs in Figure 9-5.

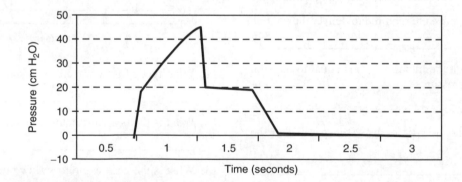

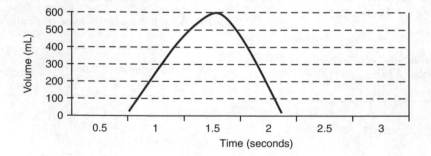

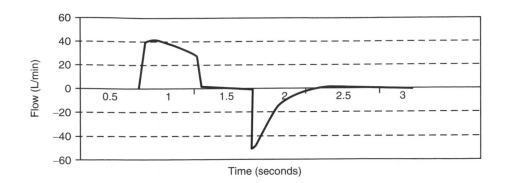

23. What is the PIP? _____

24. What is the set flow pattern and rate? _____

25. What is the tidal volume? _____

26. Calculate the static compliance.

_____

27. Calculate the airway resistance.

_____

28. Is auto-PEEP present? _____

29. Why does the flow rate drop to zero before the end of inspiration?

_____

_____

30. During PCV, the patient's lung compliance drops. How will this affect the delivered volume?

_____

31. During PC-CMV, why does flow return to zero before the end of inspiration?

_____

32. What type of flow waveform is used during PCV?

_____

33. When does the highest pressure gradient between the ventilator and the lungs occur?

_____

34. What parameters need to be set to deliver PSV?

_____

47. What is the approximate flow cycle percent in *A*?

_____

48. What is the patient tidal volume in *A*?

_____

49. What is the approximate flow cycle percent in *B*?

_____

50. What is the patient tidal volume in *B*?

_____

51. What are the approximate inspiratory times in breaths *A* and *B*?

_____

52. Why is the T_I longer for *B* than for *A*?

_____

For Questions 53 through 56, refer to the pressure-volume loop in Figure 9-10.

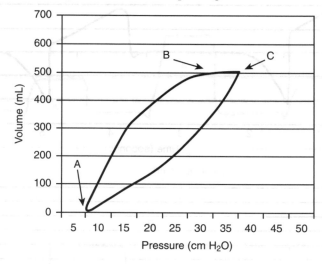

53. Identify points *A*, *B*, and *C*.

_____

54. What is the PIP?

_____

55. What is the tidal volume?

_____

56. Why does the loop begin and end at $5 \, cm \, H_2O$?

_____

57. What happens to a pressure-volume loop when lung compliance decreases during VC-CMV?

_____

58. What happens to a pressure-volume loop when lung compliance decreases during PC-CMV?

_____

59. What causes the pressure-volume loop to widen or bulge?

_____

80

For Questions 60 through 65, refer to the pressure-volume loops in Figure 9-11.

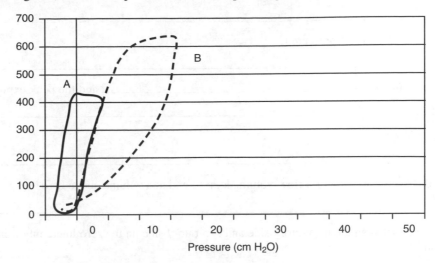

Pressure (cm H_2O)

60. What type of breath does loop *A* represent?

_____

61. In which direction does loop *A* move? Why?

_____

62. What type of breath does loop *B* represent?

_____

63. In which direction does loop *B* move? Why?

_____

64. The set flow is 45 L/min; calculate the Raw.

_____

65. The difference between the inspiratory and expiratory curves on a volume-pressure loop is called

_____.

For Questions 66 through 69, refer to the flow-volume loop in Figure 9-12.

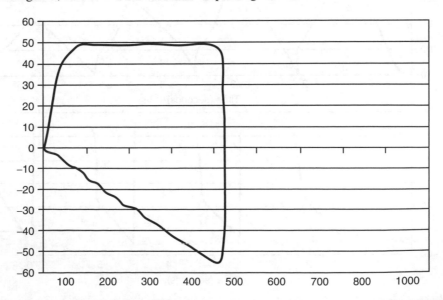

66. In which direction does this loop move?

_____

67. What type of flow waveform is represented?

_____

68. The set inspiratory flow rate is _____, and the peak expiratory flow rate is

_____.

69. What is the tidal volume?

_____

70. What can cause the expiratory side of a flow-volume loop to end at a volume above zero?

_____

71. What can cause a gap between the inspiratory side and expiratory side on the zero intercept of the y axis (flow) of a flow-volume loop?

_____

CRITICAL THINKING QUESTIONS

For Questions 1 through 8, refer to the graphs in Figure 9-13.

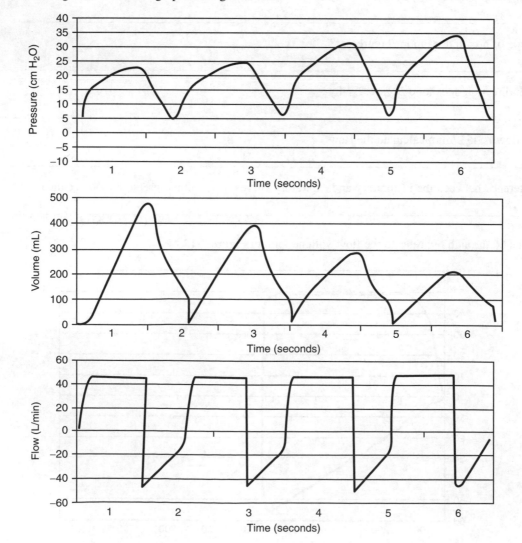

1. What mode of ventilation is being delivered?

_____

2. Is this patient assisting?

_____

3. What are the total cycle time, T_I, expiratory time, and set rate?

_____

_____

4. Describe the problem that is noticeable on the pressure-time curve.

_____

_____

_____

_____

5. Describe the two problems that are noticeable on the volume-time curve.

_____

_____

_____

_____

6. Describe the problem that is noticeable on the flow-time curve.

_____

_____

_____

_____

7. Taking into consideration the three scalars, what is causing these waveform problems?

_____

_____

_____

_____

8. What can be done to eliminate the cause of these problems?

_____

_____

_____

Case Study 1

A 68-year-old female who is 63 inches tall and weighs 120 lb was admitted through the ED with crushing chest pain. The patient has a history of COPD. Angiography was performed, and the patient subsequently underwent coronary artery bypass surgery. She now is in the cardiovascular ICU receiving mechanical ventilation. Figure 9-14 shows a current pressure-volume loop for this patient.

1. What accounts for the shape of this loop?

_____

_____

_____

_____

2. Is the patient triggering the ventilator? Explain.

_____

_____

_____

_____

3. What is the set tidal volume?

_____

_____

_____

_____

4. What is the PIP? _____

5. How should the ventilator settings be changed at this time?

_____

_____

_____

_____

_____

Case Study 2

You are the respiratory therapist in the ICU of a large municipal hospital. During rounds you note the pressure-volume loop in Figure 9-15 for one of your patients.

Pressure (cm H_2O)

1. What type of breath is represented?

_____

2. What does the portion of the loop labeled *A* represent?

_____

3. What does the portion of the loop labeled *B* represent?

_____

4. This type of loop moves in what direction?

_____

5. Has PS been set for this patient? Explain.

_____

_____

_____

_____

At the next patient-ventilator system check for this patient, you note the pressure-volume loop shown in Figure 9-16.

Pressure (cm H_2O)

6. What type of ventilatory support is the patient receiving?

_____

_____

7. Is the patient making some inspiratory effort?

_____

_____

8. What ventilator adjustment is most appropriate for this patient at this time? Why?

_____

_____

You change the graphic display and now see the graph shown in Figure 9-17.

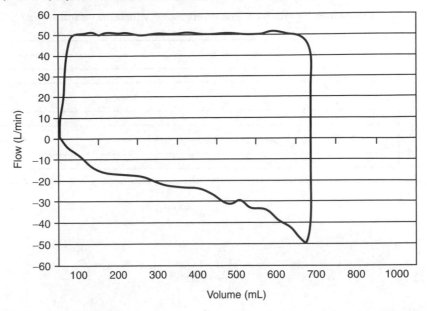

9. What data can be obtained from this loop?

_____

_____

An hour later, you receive an urgent page to come to this patient. Figure 9-18 shows the current flow-volume loop.

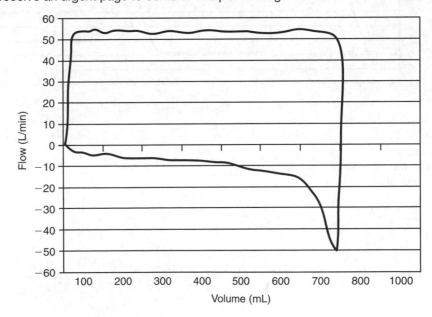

10. Explain the difference between the two flow-volume loops in Figures 9-17 and Figure 9-18.

_____

11. What is the most likely cause of this difference?

_____

12. What therapeutic intervention should you recommend for this patient?

_____

1. In the pressure-time scalar shown in Figure 9-19, line *A* represents which of the following?

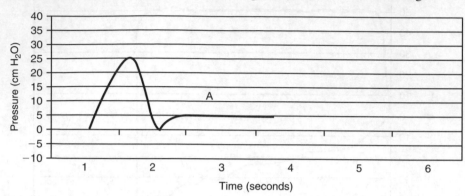

a. Auto-PEEP
b. $P_{plateau}$
c. PS
d. Transairway pressure

2. In the pressure-time scalar shown in Figure 9-20, the difference between curve *A* and curve *B* is due to which of the following?

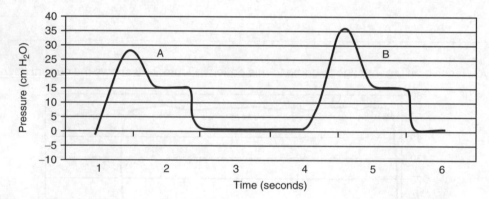

1. Atelectasis
2. Bronchospasm
3. Increased airway secretions
4. Pulmonary edema
a. 1 and 2
b. 1 and 3
c. 2 and 3
d. 2 and 4

3. Using curve *B* in Figure 9-20, calculate the Raw if the set inspiratory flow rate is 40 L/min.
   a. 0.5 cm H_2O/L/sec
   b. 2 cm H_2O/L/sec
   c. 30 cm H_2O/L/sec
   d. 52 cm H_2O/L/sec

4. The problem with the pressure-time scalar shown in Figure 9-21 is which of the following?

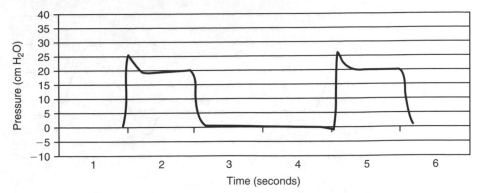

a. Patient is actively exhaling
b. Pressure rise is too rapid
c. Sensitivity setting is incorrect
d. Inspiratory pause is too long

5. Correction of the problem identified in Question 4 includes which of the following?
a. Shorten the T_I
b. Reduce the sensitivity
c. Adjust the inspiratory slope
d. Eliminate the inspiratory pause

6. During PSV for a patient with COPD, the respiratory therapist notices a pressure increase toward the end of inspiration on the pressure-time scalar. This phenomenon can be corrected by which of the following?
a. Shorten the set inspiratory time
b. Increase the flow cycle percent
c. Lower the set PS level
d. Increase the inspiratory flow setting

7. A pressure-volume loop during VC-CMV extends farther to the right and flattens out with which of the following conditions?
a. Pneumonia
b. Bronchitis
c. Asthma
d. Emphysema

8. A flow-volume loop is incomplete because the volume does not return to zero. This can be caused by which of the following conditions?
a. Air trapping
b. Flow starvation
c. Bronchopleural fistula
d. Overdistention of alveoli

Chapter **9** **Ventilator Graphics**

9. The pressure-time scalar for VC-CMV shown in Figure 9-22 demonstrates which of the following problems?

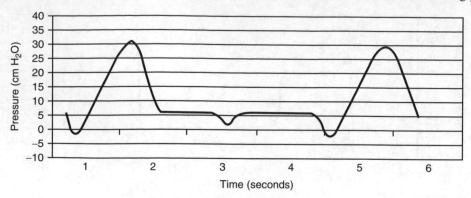

Time (seconds)

a. Flow starvation
b. Active exhalation
c. Patient-ventilator dyssynchrony
d. Incorrect sensitivity setting

10. The flow-volume loop for VC-CMV shown in Figure 9-23 demonstrates which of the following problems?

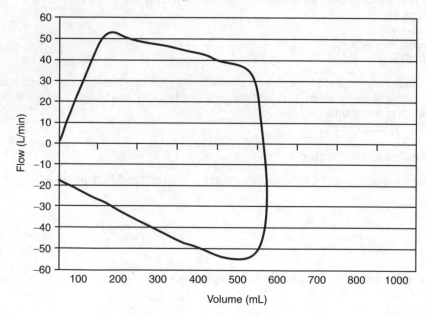

Volume (mL)

a. Atelectasis
b. Auto-PEEP
c. Flow starvation
d. Bronchopleural fistula

10 Assessment of Respiratory Function

LEARNING OBJECTIVES

Upon completion of this chapter, the reader will be able to do the following:

1. Describe the principle of operation of the pulse oximeter.
2. Identify conditions that can influence the accuracy of pulse oximetry readings.
3. Name the test used to determine disparities between arterial oxygen saturation (SaO_2), arterial oxyhemoglobin saturation (SpO_2), and the patient's clinical condition.
4. Discuss the normal components of a capnogram.
5. Give examples of pathophysiologic conditions that can alter the contour of the capnogram.
6. Identify the normal value for arterial to end-tidal partial pressure of carbon dioxide ($P[a\text{-}et]CO_2$).
7. Describe the various components of a volumetric CO_2 tracing, and discuss how these types of tracings can be used to assess gas exchange during mechanical ventilation.
8. Explain the theory of operation of transcutaneous PO_2 and PCO_2 monitors.
9. List the clinical data that should be recorded when making transcutaneous measurements.
10. Describe the major components of an indirect calorimeter.
11. Provide the respiratory quotient (RQ) value associated with substrate utilization patterns in normal, healthy subjects.
12. Discuss some clinical applications of metabolic monitoring in critically ill patients.
13. Briefly describe devices that are used to measure airway pressures, volumes, and flows during mechanical ventilation.
14. Calculate mean airway pressure, dynamic compliance, static compliance, and airway resistance.
15. Identify pathological conditions that alter lung compliance and airway resistance.
16. Describe how changes in airway resistance and respiratory system compliance will affect the results of measurements of the work of breathing.
17. Define pressure-time product, and discuss its application in the management of mechanically ventilated patients.

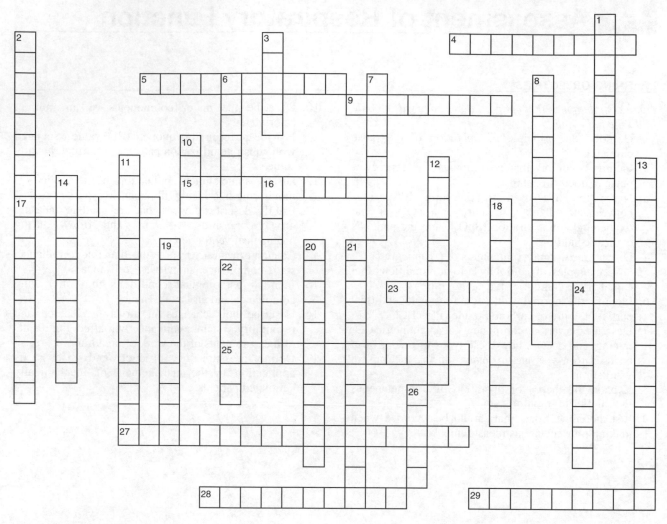

Across

4 The type of pressure measured by occluding the airway during the first 100 milliseconds of a patient's spontaneous inspiration
5 A method of sampling respired gases
9 The type of deadspace free of carbon dioxide
15 Opposition to airflow
17 The type of pressure that reflects alveolar pressure
23 A continuous, noninvasive method of assessing arterial oxygen saturation (two words)
25 Qualitative estimates of exhaled carbon dioxide are made with a _____ detector
27 Relies on the Beer-Lambert Law
28 The type of hemoglobin that is calculated by dividing the oxyhemoglobin concentration by concentration of hemoglobin capable of carrying oxygen
29 A breakdown product of heme metabolism that causes a yellow discoloration of the skin

Down

1 A factor that affects pulse oximetry readings because of movement
2 The difference between gastric and esophageal pressures
3 A common problem when monitoring at the skin surface
6 A cause of increase in the volume of carbon dioxide produced
7 An estimation of energy expenditure from measurements of oxygen consumption and carbon dioxide production is known as _____ calorimetry
8 States of low perfusion
10 Force times distance
11 Monitoring at the skin surface is known as _____ monitoring
12 A low perfusion state

Chapter **10** **Assessment of Respiratory Function**

Down—Cont'd

13 The type of hemoglobin that has carbon monoxide attached to it

14 A type of device that has an analyzer directly attached to the endotracheal tube

16 The shape of the oxyhemoglobin dissociation curve

18 The measurement of carbon dioxide concentration in respired gases

19 Lung volume achieved for a given amount of applied pressure

20 Instrument accuracy depends on this

21 Absorbs more light at 940 nm

22 Cyclical changes in light transmission allows _____ plethysmography to estimate pulse rate

24 Carbon dioxide at the end of the alveolar phase is referred to as this (hyphenated word)

26 The type of hemoglobin that absorbs both red and infrared light (abbreviation)

CHAPTER REVIEW QUESTIONS

1. List five ways of noninvasively monitoring the respiratory function of mechanically ventilated patients.

   a. _____

   b. _____

   c. _____

   d. _____

   e. _____

2. Name four causes associated with hypoxemic events in mechanically ventilated patients.

   a. _____

   b. _____

   c. _____

   d. _____

3. Name four sites where a pulse oximetry sensor may be placed.

   a. _____

   b. _____

   c. _____

   d. _____

4. The two principles on which pulse oximetry is based are _____ and

   _____.

5. How is oxyhemoglobin and deoxyhemoglobin differentiated by pulse oximetry?

   _____

   _____

   _____

   _____

6. How is pulse rate determined by a pulse oximeter?

   _____

   _____

   _____

   _____

   _____

7. What determines the accuracy of any diagnostic instrument?

   _____

8. Under what SpO_2 reading should an ABG be drawn to confirm the patient's oxygen saturation?

   _____

9. Identify four conditions that can influence the accuracy of pulse oximetry readings.

   a. _____

   b. _____

   c. _____

   d. _____

10. Name three factors that contribute to low perfusion states in patients.

    a. _____

    b. _____

    c. _____

11. The four types of hemoglobin that adult blood typically contains are:

    a. _____

    b. _____

    c. _____

    d. _____

12. What is the difference between fractional hemoglobin saturation and functional hemoglobin saturation?

_____

_____

_____

_____

13. When COHb is present in the blood what happens to the SpO_2? _____ .

14. MetHb presence in the blood is a complication of what medications?

_____

_____

15. What effect does MetHb have on SpO_2?

_____

_____

16. How does nail polish affect SpO_2?

_____

_____

17. What affect does skin pigmentation have on SpO_2?

_____

_____

18. What test is used to determine disparities between SpO_2, SaO_2, and a patient's clinical condition?

_____

_____

_____

19. The continuous display of carbon dioxide concentrations as a graphic waveform is called a

_____ .

20. In what specific clinical situation would chemical capnometer, or colorimetric detector, be particularly useful?

_____

_____

_____

21. What affect does the presence of water vapor and nitrous oxide have on the accuracy of CO_2 measurements?

_____

_____

_____

22. Describe the two methods of gas sampling used by IR analyzers.

a. _____

b. _____

23. The normal percentage of CO_2 in expired air is

_____ .

24. Identify and explain the labeled parts of Figure 10-1.

A _____

B _____

C _____

D _____

E _____

25. What determines the amount of CO_2 produced? Explain the relationship.

_____

_____

_____

26. What pathophysiologic conditions increase or decrease a patient's metabolic rate?

_____

_____

_____

27. For a normal individual, what is the relationship between $PetCO_2$ and $PaCO_2$?

_____

_____

28. What pathophysiologic conditions cause a decrease in ventilation relative to perfusion, thereby causing a higher than normal $PetCO_2$?

_____

_____

29. Where is the lowest $PetCO_2$ reading in the lungs found?

_____

_____

30. What pathophysiologic conditions cause a decrease in perfusion relative to ventilation, thereby causing a lower than normal $PetCO_2$?

_____

_____

_____

31. Name at least four pathophysiologic conditions that can alter the contour of a capnogram.

a. _____

b. _____

c. _____

d. _____

32. What do the labeled capnogram waveforms in Figure 10-2 represent?

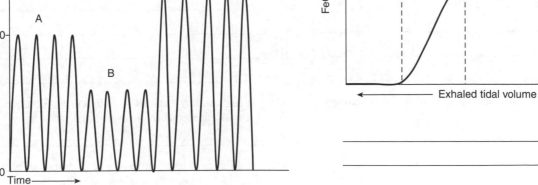

_____

_____

33. What pathological condition mimics esophageal intubation identified by capnography?

_____

_____

34. What situations may cause gastric PCO_2 to be at almost normal $PetCO_2$ levels?

_____

_____

35. Measuring the CO_2 at the end of a forced vital capacity is called the

_____

_____.

36. What should the $P(a-et)CO_2$ measurement be during normal tidal breathing?

_____

_____

37. What are the x and y axes in a volumetric CO_2 tracing?

_____

_____

38. Identify and explain the phases represented by the letters in Figure 10-3, which shows a single breath CO_2 curve.

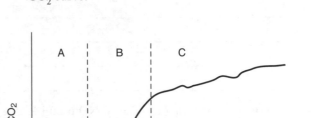

_____

_____

_____

_____

_____

39. Label all the blanks in Figure 10-4.

40. Explain the three areas of a volumetric CO_2 tracing.

a. _____

b. _____

c. _____

41. What are the four major events that influence the way CO_2 is exhaled through the lungs?

a. _____

b. _____

c. _____

d. _____

42. How can trending $\dot{V}CO_2$ be used during the weaning process?

_____

_____

_____

_____

_____

43. Why is the monitoring of exhaled NO useful in the management of severe asthma?

_____

_____

_____

44. What type of electrode is used in a transcutaneous oxygen monitor?

_____

_____

45. Why is the transcutaneous oxygen probe heated?

_____

_____

_____

_____

46. For what type of patient is transcutaneous oxygen monitoring best suited?

_____

_____

47. List five causes of erroneous $PtcO_2$ readings.

a. _____

b. _____

c. _____

d. _____

e. _____

48. What type of electrode is used for transcutaneous carbon dioxide measurements?

_____

_____

49. What affect does heating the transcutaneous carbon dioxide probe have on the measurements?

_____

_____

_____

50. How often should the transcutaneous electrode and sensor membrane be changed?

_____

_____

_____

51. What steps need to be taken when placing a transcutaneous electrode on the patient's skin?

_____

_____

_____

_____

52. The high and low values for a 2-point calibration of a transcutaneous oxygen monitor are

_____ and _____ .

53. The high and low values for a 2-point calibration of a transcutaneous carbon dioxide monitor are

_____ and _____ .

54. List the clinical data that should be documented when making transcutaneous measurements.

_____

_____

_____

_____

_____

55. How often should a transcutaneous sensor be repositioned?

_____

56. What device is most commonly used to perform indirect calorimetry?

_____

57. Describe the major components of an indirect calorimeter.

_____

_____

_____

_____

_____

_____

58. What position should the patient be in and for how long before making an indirect calorimetry measurement?

_____

_____

59. The room temperature should be between _____ and _____ when obtaining indirect calorimetry readings.

60. Why is a urinary nitrogen level necessary for calculating energy expenditure?

_____

_____

_____

61. What is the energy expenditure (EE) of a normal healthy adult?

_____

62. A hypermetabolic state exists when EE is

_____, and a hypometabolic state

exists when EE is _____.

63. Name seven conditions that cause hypermetabolic states and five conditions that cause hypometabolic states.

a. _____

b. _____

c. _____

d. _____

e. _____

f. _____

g. _____

64. What is the RQ range for a healthy adult consuming a typical American diet?

_____

65. The RQ for feedings of large amounts of glucose

is _____ and for prolonged

starvation is _____.

66. When CO_2 production increases, what happens to the respiratory quotient?

_____

67. How can diet cause a patient to fail to wean from mechanical ventilatory support?

_____

_____

_____

_____

68. The devices used to measure airway pressures in the current generation of adult and neonatal ventilators

are _____.

69. What are the most common airway pressure measurements?

_____

70. Explain how a static pressure is obtained on newer ventilators.

_____

_____

71. What factors influence plateau pressure?

_____

_____

Chapter **10** **Assessment of Respiratory Function**

2. The patient's physician asks the respiratory therapist for a recommendation as to which laboratory studies to order to clarify or confirm the pulse oximeter reading. What studies are appropriate for this patient at this time?

_____

_____

Case Study 2

A patient is brought to the emergency department following an apartment fire. The patient is brought in receiving oxygen from a nonrebreathing mask. Because there are facial burns, the patient is intubated and placed on mechanical ventilatory support with 50% oxygen. The pulse oximeter is reading 99%.

1. Is the pulse oximeter reading accurate? Why or why not?

_____

_____

An ABG analysis shows an oxygen saturation of 95% while receiving 50% oxygen.

2. Is this saturation accurate? Why or why not?

_____

_____

3. In this situation, what lab test should be suggested and why?

_____

_____

Case Study 3

A patient is in the process of being weaned from mechanical ventilatory support and is in the SIMV mode and is being monitored for end-tidal CO_2. The respiratory therapist has just decreased the ventilator rate to 4 breaths per minute; the set V_T is 500 mL. In Figure 10-5, A and B show the tracings that occurred after this change.

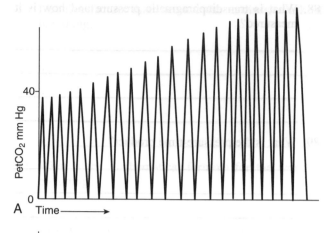

A   Time ⟶

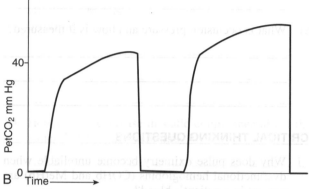

B   Time ⟶

1. Analyze both the CO_2 trend and waveform.

_____

_____

2. What are the possible causes for the CO_2 trend?

_____

_____

The respiratory therapist observes the patient using accessory muscles during spontaneous breathing. In addition there is a decreasing spontaneous tidal volume and increasing spontaneous respiratory rate.

3. How do these findings correlate with the PetCO$_2$ findings?

_____

_____

_____

4. How can the problem be alleviated?

_____

_____

Case Study 4

A respiratory therapist is monitoring the arterial to maximum end-expiratory PCO$_2$ difference for a COPD patient who is receiving mechanical ventilatory support. Over the past 24 hours, the P(a-et)CO$_2$ has increased from 5 mm Hg to 18 mm Hg.

1. Is this increase one that is expected for a patient with COPD? Why or why not?

_____

_____

2. What would a single breath CO$_2$ curve look like for this situation?

_____

_____

_____

NBRC-STYLE QUESTIONS

1. A pulse oximeter is generally considered accurate for oxygen saturations greater than which of the following?
   a. 65%
   b. 70%
   c. 75%
   d. 80%

2. A respiratory therapist encounters a patient whose pulse oximetry reading is 73%. The most appropriate action is which of the following?
   a. Change the sensor and move it to a different location.
   b. Contact the patient's physician for further instructions.
   c. Confirm the value with arterial blood CO-oximeter analysis.
   d. Accept the value and record it in the patient's medical record.

3. The response time of a pulse oximeter is most directly affected by which of the following?
   a. The type of pulse oximeter
   b. The location of the sensor or probe
   c. The percentage of oxygen saturation
   d. The position of the patient in the bed

4. The oxyhemoglobin concentration divided by the concentration of hemoglobin capable of carrying oxygen determines which of the following?
   a. Dysfunctional hemoglobin
   b. Fractional hemoglobin
   c. Functional hemoglobin
   d. Methemoglobin

5. On rounds, a respiratory therapist encounters a patient who is receiving supplemental oxygen and whose SpO$_2$ is constantly displaying 85%. The respiratory therapist notes that the patient is also receiving dapsone. The most appropriate action to take is which of the following?
   a. Use an ear lobe probe for more accuracy.
   b. Contact the patient's physician for further instructions.
   c. Confirm the value with arterial blood CO-oximeter analysis.
   d. Accept the value and record it in the patient's medical record.

6. The partial pressure of end-tidal carbon dioxide is read at what point on a capnogram?
   a. During phase 1
   b. End of phase 2
   c. During phase 3
   d. End of phase 4

7. The arterial to *maximum* expiratory PCO$_2$ gradient will be greatest for a patient with which of the following?
   a. COPD
   b. Asthma
   c. Left-heart failure
   d. Pulmonary embolism

8. The most reliable method for ruling out esophageal intubation is which of the following?
   a. Presence of CO_2 in the patient's exhaled gas
   b. Presence of condensation in the endotracheal tube
   c. Presence of bilateral breath sounds on auscultation
   d. Increased resistance to squeezing the manual resuscitator bag

9. Most likely, cardiac arrest will cause a colorimetric CO_2 detector to display which of the following?
   a. Less than 1% CO_2
   b. 1% to 2% CO_2
   c. 2% to 5% CO_2
   d. Greater than 5% CO_2

10. A respiratory therapist is called to the bedside of a patient who is being transcutaneously monitored for PO_2 and PCO_2. The signal is drifting and will not stabilize during calibration. The most appropriate action includes which of the following?
    1. Recalibrate the monitor with 15% and 20% CO_2.
    2. Clean the electrode and change the sensor membrane.
    3. Remove excess electrolyte solution from the electrode surface.
    4. Add a drop of electrolyte solution to the electrode surface.
    a. 1 and 2 only
    b. 1 and 3 only
    c. 2 and 4 only
    d. 3 and 4 only

11. A difficult to wean patient with COPD has an RQ of 0.98. The most likely cause of this patient's inability to be weaned is which of the following?
    a. Reliance on lipid metabolism is causing hypoxemia.
    b. Lipogenesis is causing the patient to retain CO_2.
    c. A highly restricted carbohydrate metabolism is generating hypoxia.
    d. Excessive carbohydrates are overloading the patient's ventilatory reserve.

12. The tracing of a slow-speed capnograph is not returning to zero every exhalation. The most likely cause of this finding is which of the following?
    a. The F_IO_2 was decreased.
    b. The patient is hyperventilating.
    c. CO_2 is being re-breathed.
    d. The capnograph needs to be re-calibrated.

13. A respiratory therapist monitoring a patient receiving mechanical ventilatory support finds that over the past two hours the patient's PIP is increasing but the static pressure has remained stable. This could be caused by which of the following?
    a. Atelectasis
    b. Pneumothorax
    c. Retained secretions
    d. Right mainstem intubation

14. Intrinsic work of breathing will be increased by which of the following?
    a. Bronchospasm
    b. Endotracheal tube
    c. Machine sensitivity
    d. Heat moisture exchanger

15. Figure 10-6 is indicative of which of the following?

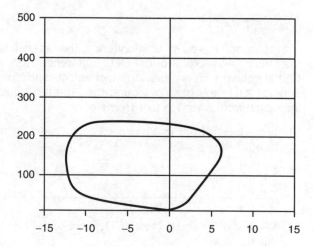

   a. Mechanical breath with little work of breathing
   b. Spontaneous breath under normal circumstances
   c. Spontaneous breath with high impedance to breathing
   d. Patient breathing through a freestanding CPAP system

11 Hemodynamic Monitoring

LEARNING OBJECTIVES

Upon completion of this chapter, the reader will be able to do the following:

1. Discuss how changes in heart rate, preload, contractility, and afterload can alter cardiac function and cardiac output.
2. Identify indicators of left ventricular preload, contractility, and afterload.
3. Name the major components of a hemodynamic monitoring system.
4. Explain the proper technique for the insertion and maintenance of a systemic arterial line, and list the most common complications that can occur with this type of monitoring system.
5. Describe the procedures for the insertion and placement of a central venous line, a balloon flotation, and a flow-directed pulmonary artery catheter; and list the potential complications associated with these devices.
6. Interpret the waveforms generated during the insertion of a pulmonary artery catheter.
7. Calculate arterial and venous oxygen content, cardiac output, cardiac index, stroke index, cardiac cycle time, left ventricular stroke work index, right ventricular stroke work index, and pulmonary and systemic vascular resistance.
8. List normal values for measured and derived hemodynamic variables.
9. Describe the most common complications associated with pulmonary artery catheterization and discuss strategies that can be used to minimize these complications.
10. Compare the effects of spontaneous and mechanical ventilation breathing on hemodynamic values.
11. Define the following terms: *incisura, pulse pressure, stroke index, stroke work, systemic vascular resistance, pulmonary vascular resistance,* and *ejection fraction.*
12. Explain how measurements of pulmonary capillary wedge pressure can be used to evaluate left ventricular function.
13. Differentiate between cardiogenic and noncardiogenic pulmonary edema using hemodynamic parameters.
14. From a patient case, describe how hemodynamic monitoring can be used in the diagnosis and treatment of selected cases of critically ill patients.

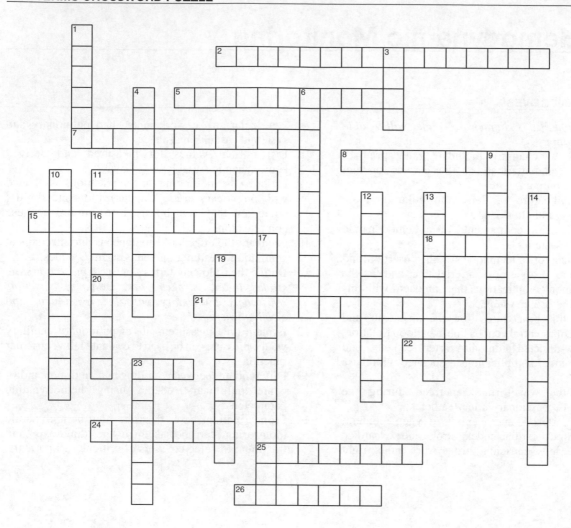

Across

2 Ratio of the stroke volume to the ventricular end-diastolic volume (two words)
5 Type of pressure exerted by fluid not moving
7 Type of pressure exerted by moving fluid
8 Flowing in the opposite direction
11 One of the atrioventricular valves
15 Slow heart rate
18 Valve between the left atrium and left ventricle
20 Left ventricle must pump against this resistance (abbreviation)
21 Type of catheter line that is inserted into the right atrium (two words)
22 Another name for pulmonary capillary wedge pressure (abbreviation)
23 The resistance that the right ventricle must pump against (abbreviation)
24 A pulmonary artery catheter floats because of this
25 Small negative deflection on the aortic and pulmonary artery tracing
26 Contraction that causes ejection of blood from the heart

Down

1 The unit for pulmonary artery catheter size
3 Principle used to calculate cardiac output
4 Quantification of the amount of pressure generated by the heart during systole (two words)
6 Rapid heart rate
9 Impedance that the left and right ventricles must overcome to eject blood into the great vessels
10 Stroke volume divided by body surface area (two words)
12 Work done by the ventricle to eject a volume of blood into the aorta (two words)
13 Both the aortic and pulmonary valves are this type of valve
14 Difference between the systolic and diastolic pressures (two words)
16 Cardiac relaxation and filling
17 Pumping strength of the heart
19 A type of electrical bridge used in pressure transducers
23 Filling pressure of the ventricle at the end of ventricular diastole

CHAPTER REVIEW QUESTIONS

1. List six common invasive hemodynamic measurements.

   a. _____

   b. _____

   c. _____

   d. _____

   e. _____

   f. _____

2. When the heart rate is 90 beats/minute, the length of one cardiac cycle is how many seconds?

   _____

3. What can cause retrograde flow in the heart?

   _____

4. Define *afterload*.

   _____

   _____

5. Left ventricular afterload must overcome what resistance?

   _____

6. Right ventricular afterload must overcome what resistance?

   _____

   _____

7. During atrial systole, which heart valves are open and which are closed?

   _____

   _____

8. Pressure exerted while a fluid is in motion is known as

   _____

   _____.

9. Pressure exerted while a fluid is not in motion is

   known as _____.

10. Where should a transducer be placed to measure accurately?

    _____

11. What happens to the pressure measurement if the transducer is (a) higher than the catheter tip and (b) lower than the catheter tip?

    a. _____

    b. _____

12. What four main factors influence the outputs of the right and left ventricle?

    a. _____

    b. _____

    c. _____

    d. _____

13. Define *preload*.

    _____

    _____

14. Describe how ventricular systole occurs.

    _____

    _____

    _____

    _____

    _____

    _____

15. What measurements are used to estimate right ventricular end-diastolic pressure and left ventricular end-diastolic pressure?

    _____

    _____

16. What do systemic vascular and pulmonary vascular resistances reflect?

    _____

    _____

17. List the major components of a hemodynamic monitoring system.

    _____

    _____

    _____

    _____

18. The mid-thoracic line of the patient is called the _____ and is used to perform a _____ on the transducer.

19. Why is positioning of the transducer important for accurate measurements?

_____

_____

_____

_____

_____

20. Explain the proper technique for the insertion and maintenance of a systemic arterial line.

_____

_____

_____

_____

_____

_____

21. What are the potential problems that could occur with an arterial catheter line?

_____

_____

22. What type of fluid is used to flush an arterial line? How fast should the flow be set?

_____

_____

23. What factors increase the risk of infection with an arterial line?

_____

_____

24. Why is prolonged or frequent flushing a problem for neonates and pediatric patients under 20 kg in weight?

_____

_____

25. List the uses for a central venous line.

_____

_____

_____

_____

26. When a central venous pressure (CVP) measurement is made at the end of ventricular diastole, what pressure does this estimate?

_____

_____

27. The veins used most for the insertion of a CVP line are _____.

28. CVP measurements are usually taken during which phase of breathing and in what position?

_____

_____

_____

29. Common problems and potential complications from CVP insertion include

_____

_____

_____

30. The normal value range for CVP is _____.

31. What are the pediatric and adult pulmonary artery catheter lengths and available sizes? How are they marked off for insertion purposes?

_____

_____

_____

32. How are clots avoided in a pulmonary artery catheter?

_____

_____

_____

33. Identify the structures, lettered *A* through *G* in Figure 11-1, on a four-channel pulmonary artery catheter.

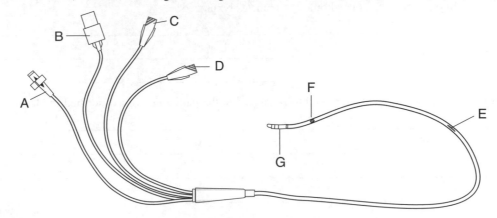

A _____

B _____

C _____

D _____

E _____

F _____

G _____

34. List the insertion sites, both percutaneous and surgical cut-down, for the insertion of a pulmonary artery catheter.

_____

_____

35. List at least eight complications associated with pulmonary artery catheterization and each cause.

a. _____

b. _____

c. _____

d. _____

e. _____

f. _____

g. _____

h. _____

36. What are the two ways to determine catheter position during insertion?

a. _____

b. _____

37. Trace the insertion of a pulmonary artery catheter from an internal jugular vein to a pulmonary vein. When is the balloon inflated? Into which lung zone should the catheter be placed?

_____

_____

_____

38. Why does the pulmonary artery catheter need to be placed in the particular zone described in Question 37?

_____

_____

_____

_____

39. What are the pressure relationships in each lung zone?

Zone	Pressure Relationship
1	_____
2	_____
3	_____

40. The volume of an adult PAC balloon is _____ and should be inflated for only _____ seconds when measuring pulmonary artery occlusion pressure (PAOP).

41. Identify the position of the catheter represented by the letters *A* through *D* in Figure 11-2.

A _____

B _____

C _____

D _____

42. How can you minimize the following common problems with pulmonary artery catheterization?

a. Ventricular arrhythmias _____

b. Pulmonary artery infarction _____

_____

c. Pulmonary artery rupture _____

d. Balloon rupture _____

43. Explain the relationship between heart rates above 200 to 220 beats/minute and a decrease in cardiac output.

_____

44. What happens to systemic arterial diastolic pressure when vasoconstriction occurs?

_____

45. Arterial systolic and diastolic pressures are affected by _____ and _____ .

46. When, in the breathing cycle, is pulmonary artery pressure measured?

_____

47. What effect does PEEP or auto-PEEP at levels above $15\,cm\,H_2O$ have on PAOP?

_____

48. Name three pathologic conditions that can alter pulmonary vascular resistance and subsequently pulmonary artery pressure.

_____

49. What does inhaled nitric oxide alter in the pulmonary vasculature?

_____

_____

50. Compare the effects of spontaneous breathing and mechanical ventilation on pulmonary artery pressure.

_____

_____

51. Complete the table below with the appropriate hemodynamic values.

Parameter	Normal Value
Arterial blood pressure	_____
Mean arterial pressure	_____
Pulse pressure	_____
Central venous pressure	_____
Pulmonary artery pressure	_____
Pulmonary artery wedge pressure	_____

52. Complete the following chart with the formulas used to calculate each value.

Calculate Value	Formula	Normal Values
Cardiac output	_____	_____
Cardiac index	_____	_____
Stroke index	_____	_____
Arterial oxygen content	_____	_____
Mixed venous oxygen content	_____	_____
Systemic vascular resistance	_____	_____
Pulmonary vascular resistance	_____	_____

Case Study 1

A 53-year-old, 6-foot-tall, 195-lb male was admitted for head trauma due to a motor vehicle accident. In the operating room, the patient had a craniotomy to relieve pressure. He is currently in the surgical intensive care unit receiving mechanical ventilation with VC-SIMV, rate 8, V_T 800 mL, F_IO_2 0.6. The patient is receiving dobutamine and nitroprusside. A pulmonary artery catheter is inserted and the following information is collected:

PAP: 38/20 mm Hg	CVP: 12 mm Hg	HR: 92 b/min
PAWP: 10 mm Hg	SBP: 145/68	Hb: 12.5 gm
CO: 5.1 L/min		

	Arterial Blood Gas	Mixed Venous Gas
pH	7.46	7.38
PCO_2	32 mm Hg	43 mm Hg
PaO_2	100 mm Hg	40 mm Hg
SaO_2	99%	75%

Calculate the following and indicate whether normal, high, or low:

1. Pulse pressure _____

2. Stroke volume _____

3. Stroke index _____

4. Cardiac index _____

5. Mean arterial pressure _____

6. Mean pulmonary artery pressure _____

7. SVR _____

8. PVR _____

9. CaO_2 _____

10. $C\overline{v}O_2$ _____

11. $C(a-v)O_2$ _____

12. DO_2 _____

13. VO_2 _____

14. RVSW _____

15. RVSWI _____

16. LVSW _____

17. LVSWI _____

18. Comment on the patient data.

_____

_____

_____

Case Study 2

The respiratory therapist is monitoring a patient who is receiving mechanical ventilatory support in one of the intensive care units. Hemodynamic monitoring of this patient is being considered because of the concern that the patient is very unstable.

1. What aspect of hemodynamic monitoring should the respiratory therapist suggest for this patient?

_____

_____

The hemodynamic monitoring system is now in place. The catheter was placed through the subclavian route about one hour ago. The patient is now exhibiting signs of respiratory distress. Breath sounds are absent on the patient's right side.

2. What complication is most likely causing this clinical situation?

_____

3. What is the most likely cause of this complication?

_____

Following correction of the problem, the PAOP was 12 mm Hg. As the day progressed, however, the pressure rose to 20 mm Hg, and then over the next few hours to 28 mm Hg. The pressure has how stabilized at 28 mm Hg.

4. What is the significance of this finding?

_____

NBRC-STYLE QUESTIONS

1. The respiratory therapist is assisting a physician inserting a pulmonary artery catheter in a patient. The respiratory therapist notes that a dampened or continuous low-pressure waveform is displayed on the oscilloscope. This indicates which of the following?
   a. The catheter is not wedged.
   b. The balloon is deflated and the catheter is not wedged.
   c. The balloon may still be inflated or the catheter may be wedged.
   d. The balloon is deflated and the catheter has perforated the right ventricle.

2. The PAOP value most indicative of cardiogenic pulmonary edema is which of the following?
   a. 8 mm Hg
   b. 12 mm Hg
   c. 18 mm Hg
   d. 25 mm Hg

3. The pressure measured from the proximal lumen of a pulmonary artery catheter is which of the following?
   a. PAP
   b. RAP
   c. RVP
   d. PAWP

4. The position of a pulmonary catheter is verified by which of the following procedures?
   a. Checking the pressure waveform
   b. Checking the number of centimeters inserted
   c. Obtaining a blood sample through the catheter tip
   d. Obtaining a chest radiograph for catheter tip placement

5. The third lumen of a pulmonary artery catheter is used to measure which of the following?
   a. CO
   b. CVP
   c. PAP
   d. PAOP

6. A low CVP value is indicative of which of the following?
   a. Shock, dehydration, or hemorrhage
   b. Shock, overhydration, or hemorrhage
   c. Hypertension, dehydration, or hypervolemia
   d. Hypertension, overhydration, and hypovolemia

7. The most common long-term complications of systemic arterial catheterization include which of the following?
   a. Hemorrhage and spasm of the artery
   b. Cardiac valve stenosis and prolapse
   c. Arterial laceration and subsequent hemorrhage
   d. Infection and tissue ischemia distal to the catheter

8. The proper location for the distal tip of a central venous catheter is in which of the following?
   a. Left ventricle or aorta
   b. Vena cava or right atrium
   c. Right ventricle or pulmonary artery
   d. Pulmonary artery or pulmonary capillary

9. Preload of the left ventricle may be estimated by which of the following measurements?
   a. RAP
   b. CVP
   c. PAP
   d. PAOP

10. Cardiac index will be increased by which of the following?
    a. Shock
    b. Exercise
    c. Hypovolemia
    d. Cardiac failure

11. Calculate the cardiac output when stroke volume is 65 mL and heart rate is 76 beats/minute.
    a. 4.9 L/min
    b. 4.6 L/min
    c. 4.5 L/min
    d. 4.3 L/min

12. Left ventricular end-diastolic volume is represented by what amount of blood?
    a. The amount ejected by the ventricle during systole
    b. The amount ejected by the ventricle during diastole
    c. The amount in the ventricle at the beginning of diastole
    d. The amount remaining in the ventricle at the end of diastole

13. While checking an indwelling CVP catheter, the respiratory therapist observes that the transducer is approximately 4 cm above the reference point. The respiratory therapist should do which of the following at this time?
    a. Add 7.44 mm Hg to the measurement.
    b. Raise the pressure transducer.
    c. Accept the CVP reading obtained.
    d. Recalibrate the pressure transducer.

14. An increase in pulmonary vascular resistance will cause which of the following?
    a. Increased right heart afterload
    b. Increased right heart preload
    c. Increased left heart afterload
    d. Increased left heart preload

15. Which of the following values indicates a patient problem?
    a. PVR = 225 dynes/sec/cm^{-5}
    b. CI = 3.8 L/min/m^2
    c. SVR = 550 dynes/sec/cm^{-5}
    d. DO_2 = 950 mL/min

12 Methods to Improve Ventilation in Patient-Ventilator Management

LEARNING OBJECTIVES

Upon completion of this chapter, the reader will be able to do the following:

1. Recommend ventilator adjustments to reduce work of breathing and improve ventilation based on patient diagnosis, arterial blood gas results, and ventilator parameters.
2. Calculate the appropriate suction catheter size, length, and amount of suction pressure needed for a specific size endotracheal tube (ET) and patient.
3. Compare the benefits of closed-suction catheters to the open suction technique.
4. Discuss the pros and cons of instilling normal saline to loosen secretions prior to suctioning.
5. List the clinical findings that are used to establish the presence of a respiratory infection.
6. Describe the procedure for prone positioning in ventilated patients with adult respiratory distress syndrome (ARDS).
7. List potential problems associated with placing the patient in a prone position during mechanical ventilation.
8. Discuss several theories that describe how prone positioning improves ventilation perfusion in ARDS.
9. Compare the protocols for using metered dose inhalers and small volume nebulizers during mechanical ventilation.
10. Describe complications associated with using small volume nebulizers powered by external flowmeters during mechanical ventilation.
11. Describe patient-centered mechanical ventilation and how it might be assessed by the respiratory therapist.
12. Discuss complications associated with the in-house transport of a mechanically ventilated patient.

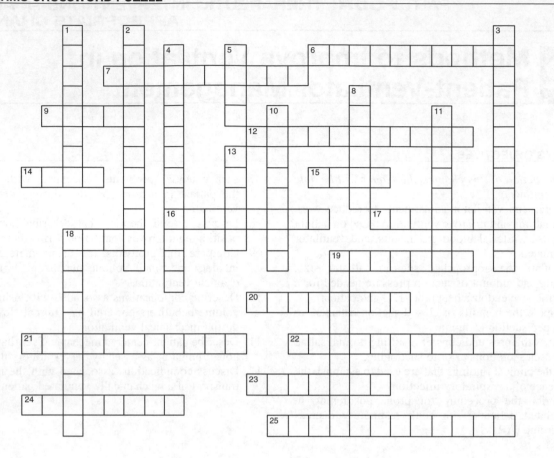

Across

6 An overdose of this will cause metabolic acidosis
7 Intentionally brought about
9 Can increase metabolism and CO_2 production
12 Normal ventilation
14 Medication given to keep pH from becoming acidotic (abbreviation)
15 Type of suctioning that can decrease VAPS in intubated patients (abbreviation)
16 CO_2 causes vasodilation here
17 Deficient blood flow to the cells
18 Type of aerosol device that delivers puffs (abbreviation)
19 A bag for collecting a patient's exhaled air
20 Rigid tonsil suction tip
21 In PCV increasing this time will increase volume delivered without increasing pressure
22 "Out of step" with the ventilator
23 A fluid filled with cellular debris and protein that accumulates as a result of inflammation
24 Respiratory acidosis indicates that this type of ventilation is not adequate
25 Part of the standard therapy to reduce increased intracranial pressure

Down

1 Reduced urinary output
2 Enteral feeding route that reduces the risks of vomiting and aspiration
3 Overhydration causes this
4 Procedure for visualizing the bronchi
5 A type of acidosis caused by diabetes, alcoholism, or starvation
8 Suctioning can cause ulceration of the _____
10 Excessive urinary output
11 Loss of bicarbonate can be caused by _____
13 A thyroid that is overactive is _____
18 Hypercapnea used to help prevent lung injury
19 Ventilation without perfusion (two words)

CHAPTER REVIEW QUESTIONS

1. Calculate the desired V_T when the known $PaCO_2$ is 55 mm Hg, the known V_T is 500 mL, the known frequency is 14, and the desired $PaCO_2$ is 40 mm Hg.

_____

_____

_____

_____

2. Calculate the desired frequency when the known $PaCO_2$ is 65 mm Hg, the known V_T is 600 mL, the known frequency is 12, and the desired $PaCO_2$ is 50 mm Hg.

_____

_____

_____

3. What three factors can affect $PaCO_2$ in patients receiving mechanical ventilation?

   a. _____

   b. _____

   c. _____

4. Identify three components of an ABG that reflect a patient's ventilatory status.

   a. _____

   b. _____

   c. _____

5. What happens to the $PaCO_2$ and pH when alveolar ventilation decreases? _____

6. List six pathologic processes that can lead to acute respiratory acidosis.

   a. _____

   b. _____

   c. _____

   d. _____

   e. _____

   f. _____

7. How does volume and pressure affect $PaCO_2$ and pH?

_____

_____

_____

8. The recommended target V_T is _____.

9. When increasing V_T it is important to maintain $P_{plateau}$ less than _____.

10. List two methods of increasing V_T in pressure-control ventilation:

    a. _____

    b. _____

11. Respiratory alkalosis is characterized by what $PaCO_2$ and pH? _____

12. List seven common causes of respiratory alkalosis:

    a. _____

    b. _____

    c. _____

    d. _____

    e. _____

    f. _____

    g. _____

13. A patient with a $PaCO_2$ of 25 mm Hg and a pH of 7.55 is sedated and ventilated in a volume-controlled mode. IBW is 60 kg. The frequency is set at 18, and the delivered V_T is set at 8 mL/kg. What frequency would result in a $PaCO_2$ of 40 mm Hg?

_____

_____

14. Is it more appropriate to change the frequency or V_T to correct a respiratory alkalosis when the delivered volume is set at 7 mL/kg? Explain your answer.

_____

_____

15. A patient on VC-CMV has the frequency set at 10, with the total respiratory rate being 20 breaths/minute. The $PaCO_2$ is 25 mm Hg with a pH of 7.52. Will decreasing the set rate correct the respiratory alkalosis? Explain your answer.

_____

_____

16. Referring to Question 15, what modes of ventilation may be more appropriate for this patient? Why?

_____

_____

17. List six common causes of hyperventilation in patients receiving mechanical ventilation:

    a. _____

    b. _____

    c. _____

    d. _____

    e. _____

    f. _____

18. What is the body's physiologic response to a metabolic alkalosis?

    _____

    _____

19. Identify six causes of metabolic alkalosis and an example of each:

    a. _____

    b. _____

    c. _____

    d. _____

    e. _____

    f. _____

20. What are the pH and bicarbonate levels that identify metabolic alkalosis?

    _____

21. What are five common causes of metabolic alkalosis?

    a. _____

    b. _____

    c. _____

    d. _____

    e. _____

22. What two formulas are needed to predict the change in pressure necessary to achieve a desired $PaCO_2$?

    a. _____

    b. _____

23. How can mechanical ventilation cause an increase in a patient's dead space?

    _____

    _____

24. Give two examples of pathologic processes that would result in an increase in physiologic dead space.

    a. _____

    b. _____

25. What is the normal range for V_D/V_T ratio?

    _____

    _____

26. Calculate the V_D/V_T ratio based on the following information: $V_T = 800\,mL$, $PaCO_2 = 45\,mm\,Hg$. $P_{\overline{E}}CO_2 = 36\,mm\,Hg$.

    _____

    _____

27. List eight clinical disorders that may result in a hypermetabolic state.

    a. _____

    b. _____

    c. _____

    d. _____

    e. _____

    f. _____

    g. _____

    h. _____

28. What effect does hyperventilation have on cerebral blood flow?

    _____

    _____

29. What is permissive hypercapnia?

    _____

    _____

30. What is the effect of permissive hypercapnia on patients with head trauma?

    _____

    _____

31. The suction pressure ranges for adults, children, and infants are:

    _____

    _____

32. The maximum length of suction time is

    _____.

33. Estimate the correct suction catheter size for a size 9.5 ET:

_____

_____

34. List at least five indications for the endotracheal suctioning of mechanically ventilated patients with artificial airways according to the AARC Clinical Practice Guidelines.

1. _____

2. _____

3. _____

4. _____

5. _____

35. What are the contraindication(s) to suctioning?

_____

_____

36. Match the complication with its most likely cause:

Complication	Cause
_____ Hypoxemia/hypoxia	a. Suction pressures
_____ Tracheal/mucosal trauma	b. Reduction in lung volume
_____ Cardiac/respiratory arrest	c. Airway trauma
_____ Cardiac arrhythmias	d. Patient or caregiver
_____ Atelectasis	e. Hypoxemia/vagal stimulation
_____ Bronchospasm	f. Extreme response to suctioning and vent disconnect
_____ Infection	g. Ventilator disconnect and loss of PEEP
_____ Bleeding	h. Reaction to tracheal stimulation

37. What are the F_IO_2 and time frame for pre- and post-suctioning hyperoxygenation?

_____

38. List the advantages and disadvantages of in-line suction catheters.

_____

_____

_____

_____

_____

_____

39. What are the high ventilator requirements that indicate the use of an in-line suction catheter?

_____

_____

40. List four reasons why silent aspiration and ventilator-associated pneumonia (VAP) can occur with cuffed ET tubes.

a. _____

b. _____

c. _____

d. _____

41. Describe how silent aspiration and ventilator-associated pneumonia occur.

_____

_____

_____

42. What is the benefit of using a Hi-Lo Evac ET tube?

_____

_____

_____

43. What pressure should be used with a CASS ET tube?

_____

44. What are some of the consequences of instilling saline prior to performing endotracheal suctioning?

_____

_____

45. How can ET suctioning be assessed while a patient is receiving mechanical ventilation?

_____

_____

_____

46. What parameters should be monitored prior to, during, and after suctioning? _____

_____

_____

47. Following suctioning of an intubated patient, the respiratory therapist notices that the sputum is rust in color. What is the patient's potential problem?

_____

48. What size suction catheter should be used for a size 4 ET tube?

_____

49. What patient-related factors influence aerosol deposition in a mechanically ventilated patient?

_____

_____

50. What are the four types of aerosol-generating devices that can be used to administer aerosolized medications during mechanical ventilation?

a. _____

b. _____

c. _____

d. _____

51. Which CMV mode is more effective for aerosol delivery?

_____

52. How do ventilator tidal volume and respiratory rate affect aerosol delivery?

_____

_____

53. What technical problems are associated with the use of SVN using an external gas source?

_____

_____

_____

54. Where, in the ventilator circuit, should the SVN, USN, and VM be placed?

_____

_____

55. What three factors would optimize the aerosol deposition of bronchodilators during noninvasive positive pressure ventilation?

a. _____

b. _____

c. _____

56. List four positive patient responses to bronchodilator therapy during mechanical ventilation.

_____

57. A mechanically ventilated patient is given albuterol via pMDI. The pre- and post-treatment findings are:
Pretreatment: PIP = $32 \, cm \, H_2O$, $P_{plateau} = 8 \, cm \, H_2O$
Post-treatment: PIP = $23 \, cm \, H_2O$, $P_{plateau} = 10 \, cm \, H_2O$
Was this treatment effective? Why or why not?

_____

_____

58. What is the goal of performing chest physiotherapy?

_____

_____

59. Chest physiotherapy includes what two procedures?

60. List the sequence of four recommended positions that aid in secretion clearance for ventilated patients:

a. _____

b. _____

c. _____

d. _____

61. List the possible hazards of performing chest physiotherapy on patients requiring mechanical ventilation:

_____

_____

62. List the three channels found in a flexible fiberoptic bronchoscope and the purpose for each:

a. _____

b. _____

c. _____

63. What medication can be given to a ventilated patient prior to a bronchoscopy to reduce secretion production and block the vagal response?

_____

64. Name three indications for the frequent changing of body position in mechanically ventilated patients.

a. _____

b. _____

c. _____

65. Placing an ARDS patient in a prone position is done for what reason?

_____

_____

66. List six mechanisms believed to improve oxygenation with prone positioning:

a. _____

b. _____

c. _____

d. _____

e. _____

f. _____

67. Match the type of contraindication with the pathologic process:

Pathologic Process

_____ Hemodynamic abnormalities

_____ Cardiac rhythm disturbances

_____ Thoracic and abdominal surgery

_____ Spinal cord instability

Contraindication

a. Absolute contraindication

b. Strong relative contraindication

c. Relative contraindication

68. What is the procedure for placing a patient in the prone position? _____

_____

69. What steps should be taken after the patient is in the prone position?

_____

_____

70. List six potential problems associated with placing a patient in a prone position.

a. _____

b. _____

c. _____

d. _____

e. _____

f. _____

71. What are the two methods of improving the ventilatory status of patients with unilateral lung disease?

a. _____

b. _____

72. What type of patient problem should be suspected when the patient's cardiac output and renal output are decreased and the PAOP is increased?

_____

73. What is normal urinary output?

_____

74. What effect can positive pressure ventilation have on urinary output?

_____

75. What effect does fluid balance have on blood cell counts?

_____

_____

_____

76. Describe the objective of patient-centered mechanical ventilation:

_____

_____

77. Which ventilator parameters can be adjusted by the respiratory therapist to improve patient comfort?

_____

_____

78. What equipment is needed for the in-house transport of a mechanically ventilated patient?

_____

_____

_____

79. What capabilities should a transport ventilator have to ensure patient safety?

_____

_____

80. Identify four contraindications to the in-house transport of a mechanically ventilated patient:

a. _____

b. _____

c. _____

d. _____

Chapter **12** **Methods to Improve Ventilation**

1. A patient is being ventilated in a volume-controlled mode. The set V_T is 700 mL with a frequency of 10. $P_{plateau}$ equals 45 cm H_2O, and the $PaCO_2$ equals 60 mm Hg. The physician would like to reduce the $PaCO_2$ to 40 mm Hg. but does not want to increase the V_T due to the high $P_{plateau}$. What can the therapist do to decrease the level of $PaCO_2$ to 40 mm Hg?

_____

_____

_____

_____

2. A post-surgical patient who suffered multiple trauma is septic with a fever of 104° F. The patient is being maintained in a volume-controlled mode of ventilation. The V_T is 800 mL, with a set frequency of 15, and the patient is triggering to 25 breaths/minute. An ABG reveals a $PaCO_2$ of 38 mm Hg, and a PaO_2 of 42 mm Hg. Why does the patient have a normal $PaCO_2$ with a minute ventilation of 20 L/min?

_____

_____

_____

_____

3. A patient in respiratory distress is intubated and placed on pressure-control ventilation with a PEEP level of +5 cm H_2O. Soon after, the patient's cardiac output decreases from 6 L/min to 4.5 L/min. What can the therapist do to help determine what was responsible for the decrease in cardiac output?

_____

_____

_____

CASE STUDIES

Case Study 1

A patient is being ventilated with VC-CMV, rate = 12 breaths/minute, V_T = 700 mL, F_IO_2 = 50%, and PEEP 5 cm H_2O. The total rate is 25 breaths/minute. The pH is 7.52, $PaCO_2$ = 30 mm Hg, and PaO_2 is 45 mm Hg. When the set frequency was reduced to 10 in an attempt to correct the respiratory alkalosis, the total rate remained at 25. An attempt at decreasing the V_T resulted in an increase in the total rate.

1. What can the therapist do to address the respiratory alkalosis for this patient?

_____

_____

_____

Case Study 2

A 100 kg (IBW) patient is receiving PCV at a set pressure of 20 cm H_2O at a frequency of 12 breaths/minute. The flow rate reaches zero before the beginning of exhalation. The exhaled volume is 550 mL, $PaCO_2$ = 65 mm Hg; pH = 7.29. The physician requests that the patient's $PaCO_2$ be decreased to 45 mm Hg.

1. What would be the most effective means of reducing the patient's $PaCO_2$?

_____

2. What parameter change would result in the desired $PaCO_2$ of 45 mm Hg?

_____

_____

_____

_____

Case Study 3

A patient with ARDS is being ventilated in a pressure-controlled mode. The PEEP level is set at 10 cm H_2O with an F_IO_2 of .60. The patient is manually ventilated with 100% O_2 prior to suctioning. When the ventilator is disconnected from the ET tube and the therapist begins the procedure, there is a rapid drop in O_2 saturation and a marked increase in the HR.

1. What is the possible cause of the problem?

_____

_____

_____

2. What can the therapist do to alleviate the situation?

_____

_____

NBRC-STYLE QUESTIONS

1. The aerosol delivery device that will affect ventilator function when used with mechanical ventilation is which of the following?
   a. pMDI
   b. USN
   c. SVN
   d. VMN

2. Permissive hypercapnia may be beneficial for a patient with which of the following?
   a. High $P_{plateau}$
   b. Intercranial lesion
   c. Pulmonary hypertension
   d. Head trauma

3. A patient requiring mechanical ventilation has an 8 mm endotracheal tube in place. The patient requires frequent suctioning and a 10 French catheter is being used. The respiratory therapist should recommend which of the following?
   a. Instill saline with every suctioning procedure
   b. A suction frequency of q2h
   c. Increase the suction pressure to -180 mm Hg
   d. Changing to a size 12 French catheter

4. Which of the following statements pertaining to the Hi-Lo Evac endotracheal tube is (are) true?
   a. The tube has a suction port at the level of the ET cuff
   b. The continuous suction pressure should be set at 30 cm H_2O
   c. The device can reduce the incidence of nosocomial pneumonias
   d. All patients should have this type of ET tube in place

5. An 85 kg male (IBW) patient is being ventilated with VC-CMV, $f = 12$ breaths/minute, $V_T = 450$ mL. The patient's ABG results reveal $PaCO_2 = 55$ mm Hg. Which of the following changes should be made to the ventilator to reduce the patient's $PaCO_2$ to 40 mm Hg?
   a. Increase the V_T to 620 mL
   b. Decrease the V_T to 400 mL
   c. Increase the rate to 18 breaths/minute
   d. Decrease the rate to 10 breaths/minute

6. A patient with a white blood cell count of 12,000 per cubic centimeter is coughing up moderate amounts of yellow secretions. Physical exam reveals decreased breath sounds and dullness to percussion. These findings are consistent with which of the following?
   a. Airway trauma
   b. Pulmonary embolism
   c. Pneumonia
   d. Pulmonary edema

7. An increase in physiologic dead space can be caused by which of the following?
   1. Pulmonary embolism
   2. An increase in V_T
   3. Low cardiac output
   4. High alveolar pressures
   a. 1 only
   b. 1 and 2
   c. 1, 3, and 4
   d. 1, 2, 3, and 4

8. A patient receiving mechanical ventilation should not be transported under which of the following conditions?
   1. Patient is hemodynamically unstable
   2. Inability to monitor cardiac function
   3. Patient is nasally intubated
   4. Patient has multiple IV lines
   a. 1 only
   b. 1 and 2
   c. 1, 3, and 4
   d. 1, 2, 3, and 4

9. Methods for managing the ventilatory status of a patient with unilateral lung disease include which of the following?
   1. Use of a double lumen endotracheal tube
   2. Instillation of normal saline prior to suctioning
   3. Bronchodilator therapy via small volume nebulizer
   4. Position the patient laterally so that the good lung is dependent
   a. 1 only
   b. 1, 2, and 3
   c. 1, 2, 3, and 4
   d. 1 and 4

10. The concept of *patient-centered mechanical ventilation* includes which of the following?
   a. Determining patient comfort level
   b. Maintaining a $PaO_2 > 60$ mm Hg
   c. Maintaining $P_{plateau} < 40$ cm H_2O
   d. Determining nutritional needs

13 Improving Oxygenation and Management of Acute Respiratory Distress Syndrome

LEARNING OBJECTIVES

Upon completion of this chapter the reader will be able to do the following:

1. Calculate a desired F_IO_2 needed to achieve a desired PaO_2, based on current ventilator settings and blood gases.
2. Calculate the pulmonary shunt fraction.
3. Identify indications and contraindications for continuous positive airway pressure (CPAP) and positive end-expiratory pressure (PEEP).
4. Name the primary goal of PEEP and the conditions in which high levels of PEEP are most often used.
5. From a PEEP study providing arterial blood gases (ABGs) and hemodynamic data, determine the optimum PEEP level.
6. Describe the most appropriate method to establish an optimum level of PEEP for a patient with acute respiratory distress syndrome (ARDS) using a recruitment-derecruitment maneuver and the deflection point (lower inflection point during deflation or derecruitment).
7. Explain what happens when a patient with a unilateral lung disease receives PEEP/CPAP therapy.
8. Describe the effects of PEEP in a patient with an untreated pneumothorax.
9. Recommend adjustments in PEEP and ventilator settings based on the physical assessment of the patient, ABGs, and ventilator parameters.
10. Compare static compliance, hemodynamic data, and ABGs as indicators of an optimum PEEP.
11. Identify from patient assessment and ABGs when it is appropriate to change from CPAP to mechanical ventilation with PEEP.
12. Define acute lung injury (ALI) and ARDS using the PaO_2/F_IO_2 ratio.
13. Recommend a tidal volume (V_T) setting in a patient with ARDS.
14. Provide the maximum $P_{plateau}$ value in patients with ARDS.
15. Identify weaning criteria from PEEP or CPAP.
16. Describe ventilator adjustments that can be performed in order to provide inverse ratio ventilation (IRV) on a conventional volume ventilator.
17. Recommend a PEEP setting based on the inflection point on the deflation curve using the pressure-volume loop for a patient with ARDS.

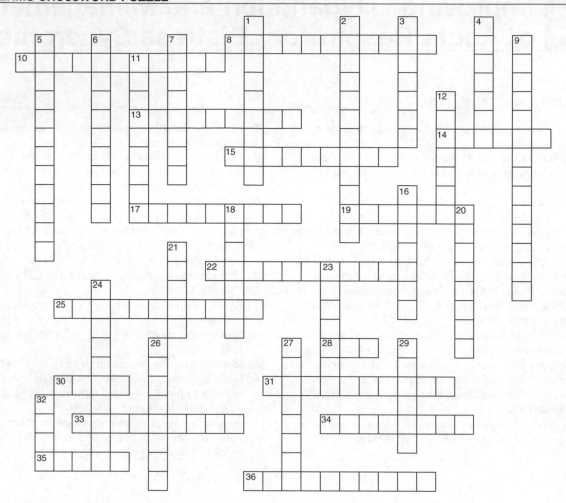

Across

8 Hemorrhaging or dehydration will cause this.
10 A maneuver used to open collapsed alveoli
13 The phase of ARDS characterized by inflammation and alveolar filling
14 Lung units
15 Point that occurs when a large number of lung units collapse quickly
17 Zone 3 of the lungs is _____.
19 The PEEP level that has maximum benefit
22 Type of pulmonary edema due to congestive heart failure (CHF)
25 Collapse of previously expanded areas of lung
28 The point on a static pressure-volume curve where the slope of the line changes significantly (abbreviation)
30 _____-billed appearance of pressure-volume curve shows overdistention.
31 Overinflation of the lungs may lead to this.
33 _____ alveolitis is the second phase of ARDS.
34 Towards the head area
35 Perfusion without ventilation
36 One type of hypoxia

Down

1 One type of inflammatory mediator
2 Creates a resistance to gas flow through an orifice (two words)
3 Alter F_IO_2 depending on oxygen saturation
4 Pressure that pulls fluid out of tissues
5 High thoracic pressures can reduce this (two words).
6 Material produced by type II pneumocytes
7 Has blood flowing through its capillaries
9 Keep F_IO_2 low to avoid this (two words).
11 A resistor that maintains pressure independent of flow
12 Pressure used to calculate static compliance
16 Material that some CPAP masks are made from
18 Type of pressure-volume loop obtained during gas flow
20 Chemical that causes inflammation
21 A Drager ventilator
23 A Hamilton ventilator
24 Point that occurs where a large number of lung units collapse quickly
26 Cellular death
27 Breath sound indicative of pulmonary edema
29 Towards the base of the spine
32 A specific clinical disorder that benefits from PEEP (abbreviation)

CHAPTER REVIEW QUESTIONS

1. Explain the difference between hypoxemia and hypoxia.

_____

_____

_____

2. What information does the measurement of oxygen delivery provide?

_____

_____

_____

3. What are the formulas for calculating oxygen delivery and consumption?

_____

_____

_____

4. How often should the F_IO_2 be monitored on adult and pediatric patients receiving mechanical ventilation?

_____

_____

5. How soon after a change in F_IO_2 is made can an ABG be drawn?

_____

6. At what level should the F_IO_2 be maintained to help prevent the complications of oxygen toxicity?

_____

7. By what mechanism can breathing 100% oxygen contribute to hypoxemia?

_____

_____

8. What is the target range for PaO_2 when administering supplemental oxygen for a non-COPD patient?

_____

9. What conditions need to be present for there to be a linear relationship between PaO_2 and F_IO_2?

_____

10. What formula is used to calculate the desired F_IO_2 necessary to obtain a desired PaO_2?

_____

11. Thirty minutes after initiating pressure-targeted ventilation an ABG is drawn with the following results: pH = 7.43, $PaCO_2$ = 43 mm Hg, PaO_2 = 50 mm Hg. The F_IO_2 is set at 75%, with a PEEP level of 5 cm H_2O. What F_IO_2 is needed to achieve a desired PaO_2 of 60 mm Hg?

_____

_____

12. What is the significance of calculating pulmonary shunt?

_____

_____

13. What is the equation for the calculation of pulmonary shunt?

_____

_____

14. Given the following information, calculate the pulmonary shunt fraction : $Cc'O_2$ = 20.4 vol%, CaO_2 = 19.8 vol%, $C\overline{v}O_2$ = 13.4 vol%

_____

_____

_____

15. Define Paw:

_____

_____

_____

16. List the factors that affect Paw during positive pressure ventilation (PPV):

_____

_____

_____

17. How does increasing Paw increase PaO_2 in the presence of ventilation/perfusion abnormalities and/or diffusion defects?

_____

18. List three methods of increasing Paw:

a. _____

b. _____

c. _____

46. Based on the following table, what is the optimal PEEP level? Explain your answer.

PEEP (cm H_2O)	PaO_2 (mm Hg)	CO (L/min)	PvO_2 (mm Hg)	C_S (mL/cm H_2O)
+3	50	3.5	27	25
+7	75	4.0	30	30
+11	90	4.5	35	37
+17	95	4.3	32	35
+22	105	4.0	30	33

_____

_____

_____

_____

_____

47. Why is PEEP therapy not beneficial to patients with emphysema?

_____

_____

48. Give an example of a nontherapeutic indication for low PEEP therapy:

_____

_____

49. Why is hypovolemia a relative contraindication for PEEP therapy?

_____

_____

50. What increments should be used to increase PEEP during a PEEP study?

_____

51. During volume-controlled ventilation, the PEEP level is set at +5 cm H_2O and the P_{peak} is 42 cm H_2O. After the PEEP is increased to 10 cm H_2O, the P_{peak} is now measured at 48 cm H_2O. Has the patient's condition worsened? What caused the increase in P_{peak}?

_____

_____

_____

52. Look at Table 13-7 in the textbook. Why was there no significant improvement in PaO_2 until the level of PEEP was increased to 15 cm H_2O?

_____

_____

53. List five uses for PEEP other than ALI:

a. _____

b. _____

c. _____

d. _____

e. _____

54. List five criteria that may indicate that a patient is ready for a trial reduction of PEEP:

   a. _____

   b. _____

   c. _____

   d. _____

   e. _____

55. Define adult respiratory distress syndrome:

   _____

   _____

   _____

56. How is ALI distinguished from the ARDS?

   _____

   _____

   _____

57. What is the difference between overdistention and hyperinflation?

   _____

   _____

   _____

58. Why is ARDS considered a systemic syndrome and not just a problem confined to the lung?

   _____

   _____

   _____

59. How does cardiogenic pulmonary edema differ from the pulmonary edema associated with ARDS?

   _____

   _____

   _____

60. What effect does ALI/ARDS have on compliance and lung volumes?

   _____

   _____

61. Identify the two phases of ARDS and the characteristics of each:

   a. _____

   b. _____

62. Describe the two categories of ARDS.

   a. _____

   b. _____

63. Why is the use of tidal volumes of 10 to 15 mL/kg no longer suggested when ventilating ARDS patients?

   _____

   _____

   _____

64. What is the goal of utilizing lung-protective strategies when ventilating a patient with ARDS?

   _____

   _____

   _____

65. What are the basic points that should be kept in mind when managing ventilated patients with ARDS using an open-lung or lung-protective strategy?

   _____

   _____

   _____

   _____

66. What conditions should be ruled out prior to performing a recruitment maneuver?

   _____

   _____

   _____

67. What is the purpose of performing a slow or static pressure ventilation (PV) loop?

   _____

   _____

   _____

68. How are the inflation and deflation portions of the PV loop utilized?

   _____

   _____

   _____

69. What is the purpose of the reinflation with a Super Syringe that is performed during a recruitment maneuver?

   _____

   _____

Chapter **13** **Improving Oxygenation and Management of ARDS**

70. What is the difference between a static PV loop and a quasi-static PV loop?

_____

_____

71. A lung recruitment maneuver provides the following information: lower inflection point on the inspiratory limb = $10\,cm\,H_2O$, upper inflection point on the inspiratory limb = $20\,cm\,H_2O$, and the upper inflection point on the deflation (UIPd) portion of the curve is $5\,cm\,H_2O$. What should the PEEP be set at and why?

_____

_____

_____

72. To avoid overdistention in the patient from the previous question, PIP should not exceed what pressure?

_____

73. Give at least three examples of types of lung recruitment maneuvers:

a. _____

b. _____

c. _____

74. An ARDS patient is on pressure-controlled continuous mandatory ventilation (PC-CMV) at a rate of 10 breaths/minute; I:E 1:1, PC is set at $20\,cm\,H_2O$ above PEEP, and PEEP is $10\,cm\,H_2O$. Describe how manipulating the PEEP level may be used to establish an optimum PEEP level for this patient:

_____

_____

_____

_____

_____

_____

Use the following table to answer questions 75 and 76.

Time	0800	0805	0810	0815	0820	0825	0830	0835	0840	0845
PEEP ($cm\,H_2O$)	0	5	10	15	20	25	30	35	40	35
C_s ($mL/cm\,H_2O$)	27	27	27	29	32	36	38	41	40	40

Time	0850	0855	0900	0905	0910	0915	0920	0925	0930	0935
PEEP ($cm\,H_2O$)	32.5	30	27.5	25	22.5	20	17.5	15	12.5	10
C_s ($mL/cm\,H_2O$)	40	38	38	38	38	37	37	28	28	27

75. At what time, PEEP level, and static compliance (C_S) did the UIPd point occur?

_____

76. What is the appropriate PEEP setting for this patient?

_____

CRITICAL THINKING QUESTIONS

1. Use the following PV loop to answer questions a through c.

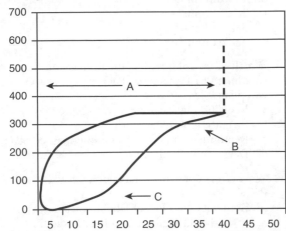

a. Identify the following points in the pressure-volume curve:

   Point A _____

   Point B _____

   Point C _____

b. Identify the point at which the lungs are overstretched:

   _____

   _____

c. Identify the point that may correlate with an increase in PaCO$_2$:

   _____

   _____

   _____

2. The following volume-pressure curve was obtained from a patient receiving volume-controlled ventilation:

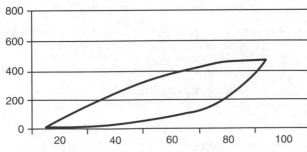

a. What is the approximate PIP?

   _____

b. What is the approximate exhaled V$_T$?

   _____

c. By observing this volume-pressure curve, can it be determined if the high airway pressure was caused by a decrease in compliance or by an increase in airway resistance?

   _____

   _____

   _____

3. A patient with ARDS and refractory hypoxemia is being ventilated in a volume-control mode. The physician would like to institute an inverse I:E ratio. What ventilatory parameters could the therapist recommend to achieve an inverse ratio in a volume mode of ventilation?

   _____

   _____

   _____

CASE STUDIES

Case Study 1

A 38-year-old patient is admitted to the emergency department and placed on volume-controlled mechanical ventilation for aspiration pneumonia.

A postextubation radiograph reveals that the endotracheal tube is in proper position. There is complete opacification of the right lung. The left lung appears normal. The peak inspiratory pressure = 62 cm H$_2$O; P$_{plateau}$ = 55 cm H$_2$O. Ventilator settings and ABG results are as follows:

Mode	VC-CMV	pH	7.43
F$_I$O$_2$	1.0	PaCO$_2$	38 torr
Frequency	20	PaO$_2$	40 torr
V$_T$	800 mL	HCO$_3$	23 mEq/L
PEEP	15 cm H$_2$O	BE	0 mEq/L

1. What could be causing the severe hypoxemia?

   _____

   _____

2. What should the therapist recommend?

   _____

   _____

Chapter **13** Improving Oxygenation and Management of ARDS

Case Study 2

A 26-year-old male is 5 ft 6 in tall and weighs 56.8 kg (125 lb). He was admitted for a heroin overdose, and was intubated and placed on volume-controlled ventilation. Chest radiograph reveals bilateral "fluffy" infiltrates. Ventilatory data and ABGs are as follows:

Mode	VC-SIMV	pH	7.37
F_IO_2	1.0	$PaCO_2$	43 torr
Frequency	12	PaO_2	44 torr
V_T	600 mL	SaO_2	85%
PEEP	5 cm H_2O	HCO_3	23 mEq/L
PIP	55 cm H_2O	BE	0 mEq/L
$P_{plateau}$	48 cm H_2O		

1. Interpret the ABG:

_____

2. What is the significance of the $P_{plateau}$?

_____

_____

3. What should the therapist recommend to treat the hypoxemia and high ventilating pressures?

_____

_____

NBRC-STYLE QUESTIONS

1. By what mechanism does PEEP cause an increase in intracranial pressure?
   a. Cardiac output and venous return are increased.
   b. Stroke volume is decreased.
   c. There is an increase in central venous pressure.
   d. Venous return is decreased, which results in intracranial hemorrhage.

2. Which of the following is an absolute contraindication to the use of PEEP or CPAP therapy?
   a. Increased intracranial pressure
   b. Severe hyperventilation
   c. Decreased lung compliance
   d. Untreated pneumothorax or tension pneumothorax

3. A 35-year-old patient diagnosed with ARDS is receiving pressure-controlled mechanical ventilation. Based on ABG results, the PEEP is increased from 14 cm H_2O to 18 cm H_2O. Which of the following should the therapist monitor immediately after making the change?
   a. Cardiac output
   b. Creatinine
   c. Hemoglobin
   d. Serum potassium

4. If the total arterial content of oxygen (CaO_2) equals 16.94 vol%, and the cardiac output (CO) is 12.54 L/min, how much oxygen is being delivered?
   a. 1000 mL/min
   b. 2.124 L/min
   c. 3.450 L/min
   d. 3.926 L/min

5. Which of the following is the primary mechanism by which PEEP increases PaO_2 and improves compliance?
   a. Reduction in mean airway pressure
   b. Increase in minute ventilation
   c. Recruitment and distension of collapsed alveoli
   d. Decrease in cardiac output

6. What effect does PEEP have on both PaO_2 and $PaCO_2$?
   a. Both PaO_2 and $PaCO_2$ should increase.
   b. PaO_2 should increase and $PaCO_2$ should decrease.
   c. Both PaO_2 and $PaCO_2$ should decrease.
   d. $PaCO_2$ should remain unaffected and PaO_2 should increase.

7. Which of the following is a direct lung insult that can result in ARDS?
   1. Pneumonia
   2. Aspiration
   3. Sepsis
   4. Smoke inhalation
   a. 1 only
   b. 1 and 2
   c. 1, 2, and 4
   d. 1, 2, 3, and 4

8. Which of the following conditions is a potential complication when instituting PEEP therapy?
   1. Decrease in cardiac output
   2. Barotrauma
   3. Altered cardiac function
   4. Decrease in urine output
   a. 1 only
   b. 3 and 4
   c. 1, 3, and 4
   d. 1, 2, 3, and 4

9. What could be the most likely cause of an increased $PaCO_2$ after an increase in the level of PEEP?
   a. Tension pneumothorax
   b. Lung overdistention
   c. An increase in compliance
   d. A decrease in airway resistance

10. When managing a patient with ARDS receiving mechanical ventilation + PEEP, what can be done to help alleviate the problem of excessive lung water?
    a. Ventilate with large tidal volumes.
    b. Increase the amount of IV fluids.
    c. Patients should be placed on diuretic therapy.
    d. Keep peak inspiratory pressures below 50 cm H_2O.

Ventilator-Associated Pneumonia

LEARNING OBJECTIVES

Upon completion of this chapter the reader will be able to do the following:

1. Define *ventilator-associated pneumonia* (VAP) and *hospital-acquired pneumonia* (HAP).
2. Differentiate between early-onset VAP and late-onset VAP and describe the overall incidence of VAP.
3. Discuss the prognosis, including morbidity and mortality rates, for patients diagnosed with VAP.
4. Identify the most common pathogenic microorganisms associated with VAP.
5. List nonpharmacologic and pharmacologic therapeutic interventions that have been shown to increase the risk of development of VAP.
6. Describe the sequence of events that are typically associated with the pathogenesis of VAP.
7. Discuss the advantages and disadvantages of using clinical findings versus quantitative diagnostic techniques to identify patients with VAP.
8. Briefly describe the criteria for starting empiric antibiotic therapy for patients without evidence of multidrug-resistant (MDR) infections and for those patients with risk of developing MDR infections.
9. Define *deescalation of antibiotic therapy* and how it can be used to reduce the emergence of MDR pathogens.
10. Discuss how *ventilator bundles* can be used to prevent VAP and the emergence of MDR pathogens in the clinical setting.

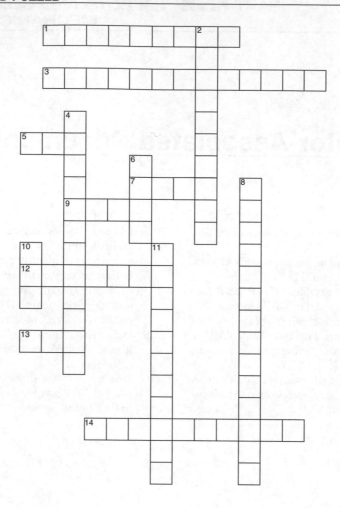

Across

1 VAP that develops later than 72 hours following tracheal intubation
3 Infection by multiple pathogenic microorganisms
5 Pathogens resistant to certain antibiotics
7 A major complication of VAP
9 An assessment criteria including fever, leukocyte count, tracheal secretion characteristics, and oxygenation status
12 Guidelines for the management of adults with HAP, VAP, and HCAP
13 Pneumonia that develops 48 hours after a patient has been placed on mechanical ventilation
14 Infection aquired in the health care setting

Down

2 VAP that develops between 48 and 72 hours following tracheal intubation
4 Used to obtain cultures from the lower respiratory tract
6 Continuous aspiration of subglottic secretions
8 Prolonged antibiotic used to ICU patients may favor selection with resistant organisms responsible for this
10 Bronchial alveolar lavage
11 Common respiratory infection seen in patients with cystic fibrosis

CHAPTER REVIEW QUESTIONS

1. Ventilatory-associated pneumonia is most often caused by what organism?

   _____

2. What are the two classifications of VAP? Describe the differences.

   a. _____

   b. _____

3. What are some common gram-negative anaerobes isolated from nosocomial pneumonias?

   _____

   _____

   _____

4. What are some common gram-positive aerobes isolated from nosocomial pneumonias?

   _____

   _____

5. What is the mortality rate range caused by VAP?

   _____

6. Guidelines for the management of patients with VAP focus on:

   _____

   _____

   _____

7. What is the most common nosocomial infection encountered in the intensive care unit?

   _____

8. The incidence of VAP for all intubated patients ranges between what percentages?

   _____

9. List at least five causes of VAP:

   a. _____

   b. _____

   c. _____

   d. _____

   e. _____

10. List at least 10 host-related factors that may increase the development of VAP in a patient:

    a. _____

    b. _____

    c. _____

    d. _____

    e. _____

    f. _____

    g. _____

    h. _____

    i. _____

    j. _____

11. What type of patients are typically at highest risk for the development of VAP?

    _____

12. Ventilated patients with chronic obstructive pulmonary disease (COPD) are susceptible to what VAP causing pathogens?

    _____

    _____

    _____

13. Ventilated patients with cystic fibrosis are more susceptible to what VAP causing pathogens?

    _____

    _____

14. VAP is a major complication of and increases the mortality rate for patients with what respiratory condition?

    _____

15. List at least four common risk factors for the development of multi-drug resistant infections:

    a. _____

    b. _____

    c. _____

    d. _____

Chapter **14** Ventilator-Associated Pneumonia

16. List at least six nonpharmacologic interventions that are associated with the increased risk of VAP:

    a. _____

    b. _____

    c. _____

    d. _____

    e. _____

    f. _____

17. List four pharmacologic interventions that can lead to the development of VAP:

    a. _____

    b. _____

    c. _____

    d. _____

18. Describe briefly the sequence of events that lead to VAP:

    _____

    _____

19. What are the six clinical assessments of the Clinical Pulmonary Infection Score (CPIS) criteria?

    a. _____

    b. _____

    c. _____

    d. _____

    e. _____

    f. _____

20. What happens to the oropharyngeal flora of invasively ventilated, critically ill patients?

    _____

21. When using all six criteria of the CPIS, what score indicates evidence of the presence of VAP?

    _____

22. What procedure has been shown to significantly improve the diagnosis of VAP?

    _____

23. What is the difference between clinical assessment (qualitative) and quantitative diagnosis of VAP?

    _____

24. The most important nonpharmacologic prevention strategy to reduce the risk of clinicians transmitting infectious microorganisms from one patient to another is what?

    _____

25. What are some ways to reduce aspiration of gastric contents?

    _____

    _____

26. What is a common pathogen associated with percutaneous tracheostomy?

    _____

27. To lessen the risk of VAP, when should ventilator circuits be changed?

    _____

    _____

28. List four pharmacologic interventions to help reduce the risk of VAP:

    a. _____

    b. _____

    c. _____

    d. _____

29. List four quantitative techniques used to diagnose VAP:

    a. _____

    b. _____

    c. _____

    d. _____

30. Successful treatment of VAP requires what two types of assessments?

    a. _____

    b. _____

31. What position should a ventilated patient be in to reduce the incidence of aspiration?

    _____

32. Why does oral intubation pose less of a risk for VAP than nasal intubation?

    _____

33. Pharmacologic and non pharmacologic strategies to reduce the incidence of VAP are incorporated into evidence-based practices known as:

    _____

CRITICAL THINKING QUESTIONS

1. A 69-year-old male patient with a history of COPD is intubated and is receiving mechanical ventilation due to trauma sustained in a motor vehicle collision. What are some factors that put this patient at an increased risk for developing ventilator-associated pneumonia and what can the therapist do to reduce this risk?

_____

_____

_____

_____

2. Why is a patient's past medical history important when determining antibiotic therapy?

_____

CASE STUDIES

Case Study 1

A patient with a history of cystic fibrosis develops a fever with purulent tracheobronchial secretions 4 days after endotracheal intubation and mechanical ventilation. The respiratory therapist suspects VAP.

1. What type of VAP is likely?

_____

2. Considering the patient's past medical history, what is the most likely pathogen causing the pneumonia?

_____

3. What can be done to diagnosis the pathogen?

_____

NBRC–STYLE QUESTIONS

1. Ventilator-associated pneumonia is most commonly caused by which of the following?
   a. Viral infection
   b. Fungal infection
   c. Bacterial infection
   d. Acute respiratory distress syndrome

2. With regard to ventilator-associated pneumonia, COPD patients are at increased risk from which of the following pathogenic organisms?
   a. *Haemophilus influenza*
   b. *Candida albicans*
   c. *Klebsiella pneumoniae*
   d. *Pseudomonas aeruginosa*

3. Therapeutic interventions that can lead to the development of ventilator-associated pneumonia include which of the following?
   a. Inappropriate antimicrobial therapy
   b. Frequent arterial blood gas analysis
   c. NIV
   d. Semirecumbent positioning of the patient

4. Independent factors that contribute to the development of ventilator-associated pneumonia include which of the following?
   1. Alcoholism
   2. Proper oral care
   3. Acidosis
   4. Acute respiratory distress syndrome
   a. 1 and 3
   b. 1 and 2
   c. 3 and 4
   d. 2 and 4

5. What is the nonpharmacologic intervention most associated with VAP?
   a. Frequent changing of the ventilator circuit
   b. Use of an ET or tracheostomy during mechanical ventilation
   c. Use of bronchoscopes
   d. Reusable ventilator probes

6. During critical illness, the shift in the normal flora of the oropharyngeal tract to gram-negative bacilli and *S. aureus* may be due to which of the following factors?
   1. Comorbidities
   2. Malnutrition
   3. Decreased airway pH
   4. Decreased production of proteases
   a. 1 and 3
   b. 1 and 2
   c. 3 and 4
   d. 2 and 4

7. Inappropriate use of what intervention is associated with the emergence of MDR pathogens?
   a. Noninvasive positive-pressure ventilation (NIV)
   b. Antibiotics
   c. Tracheostomy tubes
   d. Fiberoptic bronchoscopy

8. Which of the following refers to the process of focusing the types and duration of antibiotics used to treat VAP?
   a. Broad-spectrum antibiotic therapy
   b. Ventilator bundles
   c. Nonpharmacologic interventions
   d. Deescalating antibiotic therapy

Chapter **14** **Ventilator-Associated Pneumonia**

15 Sedatives, Analgesics, and Paralytics

LEARNING OBJECTIVES

Upon completion of this chapter the reader will be able to do the following:

1. List the most common sedatives and analgesics used in the treatment of critically ill patients.
2. Discuss the indications, contraindications, and potential side effects of each of the sedatives and analgesic agents reviewed.
3. Describe the most common method of assessing the need for and level of sedation.
4. Describe the Ramsay scale.
5. Discuss the advantages and disadvantages of using benzodiazepines, neuroleptics, anesthetic agents, and opioids in the management of mechanically ventilated patients.
6. Discuss the mode of action of depolarizing and nondepolarizing paralytics.
7. Explain how the train-of-four method is used to assess the level of paralysis in critically ill patients.
8. Contrast the indications, contraindications, and potential side effects associated with using various types of neuromuscular blocking agents (NMBAs).
9. Recommend a medication for a mechanically ventilated patient with severe anxiety and agitation.

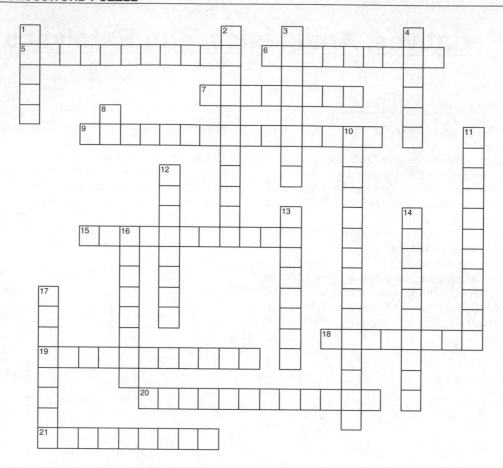

Across

5 Type of amnesia related to the prevention of new memories
6 Facilitates invasive procedures by preventing movement
7 Anesthetic agent
9 A neuromuscular blocking agent
15 Method of assessing the level of sedation (two words)
18 A benzodiazepine drug
19 Method of monitoring the depth of paralysis with an electrical current (three words)
20 Agent that resembles acetylcholine in chemical structure
21 Drug of choice for sedating mechanically ventilated patients for longer than 24 hours

Down

1 An opioid receptor
2 Haloperidol is included in this category of drugs.
3 An opioid antagonist
4 Pinpoint pupils
8 An opioid receptor
10 Agent that inhibits the action of acetylcholine at the neuromuscular junction
11 A nondepolarizing NMBA
12 Agent that reduces anziety and agitation
13 Disorganized thought patterns and excessive, nonpurposeful motor activity
14 Reverses the effects of benzodiazepines
16 A naturally occurring opioid
17 Opioid narcotic that is stronger than morphine

1. What effects do sedatives have on the body?

   _____

2. Why is paralysis used during mechanical ventilation?

   _____

3. List the four types of pharmacological agents used for sedation in the ICU. Give at least one example of each.

   a. _____

   b. _____

   c. _____

   d. _____

4. What modes of ventilation often require patients to be sedated?

   _____

5. Name the four JCAHO-defined levels of sedation.

   a. _____

   b. _____

   c. _____

   d. _____

6. Complete the following table using the four JCAHO-defined levels of sedation. What type of patient response and ventilatory and cardiovascular function do patients have at each level of sedation?

Sedation Level	Patient Response	Ventilatory Function	Cardiovascular Function

7. What level of sedation may be necessary when a patient's breathing is asynchronous with the mechanical ventilatory mode?

   _____

8. What level of sedation is necessary during weaning from mechanical ventilation?

   _____

9. What scoring systems may be used to assess the level of sedation in adults and children?

   _____

Use the Scoring System in Table 15-1 of the textbook to answer questions 10 through 12.

10. What range of scores indicates adequate sedation?

   _____

11. What score indicates the need for sedation?

   _____

12. What scores indicate oversedation of a patient?

   _____

13. Why are benzodiazepines the drugs of choice for the treatment of anxiety in critical care?

   _____

   _____

14. What is the mode of action for benzodiazepines?

   _____

   _____

   _____

   _____

15. What factors alter the intensity and duration of action of various benzodiazepines?

   _____

   _____

16. What pathological processes prolong recovery from treatment with benzodiazepines?

   _____

17. Why does diazepam have a rapid onset of action?

   _____

   _____

   _____

18. How is diazepam administered?

   _____

   _____

19. Acutely agitated patients are best treated with which benzodiazepine? Why?

   _____

   _____

20. How can prolonged sedation occur with midazolam?

   _____

   _____

   _____

21. Which benzodiazepine is best suited for sedating mechanically ventilated patients in the ICU for longer than 24 hours?

_____

22. An overdose of benzodiazepines may be reversed with what drug?

_____

23. Potential side effects of continual use of lorazepam (Ativan) include:

_____

24. What class of drugs is routinely used to treat extremely agitated and delirious patients in the ICU?

_____

25. The drug most often used to treat ICU delirium is _____.

26. What are some of the side effects of the drug in the previous question?

_____

_____

_____

27. The anesthetic agent that has proved useful for sedation of neurosurgical patients is _____.

28. What are the hemodynamic effects of the drug in the previous question?

_____

_____

29. Referring to the drug from the previous two questions, what are the advantages and disadvantages of using this drug to sedate neurological patients?

Disadvantages	Advantages
_____	_____
_____	_____
_____	_____
_____	_____
_____	_____
_____	_____

30. Name the two most commonly used opioids:

    a. _____

    b. _____

31. List three effects that opiates have on the body.

    a. _____

    b. _____

    c. _____

    d. _____

Chapter **15** **Sedatives, Analgesics, and Paralytics**

32. How do opiates exert their effects on the body?

_____

_____

33. List at least ten side effects of opioids.

a. _____

b. _____

c. _____

d. _____

e. _____

f. _____

g. _____

h. _____

i. _____

j. _____

34. What determines the severity of the side effects of opioids?

_____

35. Which drug can reverse the respiratory depression caused by opioids?

_____

36. What effects does morphine have on the central nervous system?

_____

_____

_____

37. How does morphine affect the gastrointestinal tract?

_____

_____

_____

38. How does morphine affect the cardiovascular system?

_____

_____

39. Which opioid should be used for a patient whose hemodynamic status is unstable?

_____

40. Complete the following table.

	Morphine	Fentanyl
Is it natural or synthetic?	_____	_____
Is it lipid soluble?	_____	_____
Does it cross the blood-brain barrier?	_____	_____
What is the onset of action?	_____	_____
What is the duration of action?	_____	_____
How is it administered?	_____	_____

41. Increased intracranial pressure caused by traumatic brain injury may be controlled by a combination of which two drugs?

_____

42. What type of drug is used to reduce oxygen consumption and carbon dioxide production?

_____

43. What is the difference between depolarizing and nondepolarizing agents?

_____

44. Why are NMBAs used while a patient is being mechanically ventilated?

_____

_____

_____

45. What is the purpose of train-of-four monitoring (TOF)?

_____

46. How does TOF operate?

_____

_____

47. According to the Society for Critical Care Medicine, what indicates that an adequate amount of NMBA is being administered when TOF is used?

_____

48. What other medication is necessary when a paralytic agent is used?

_____

_____

49. The most widely used depolarizing NMBA is:

_____

50. What are the onset of action and duration of action for the drug referred to in question 49?

_____

51. For what purpose is the drug referred to in question 49 used?

_____

Chapter **15** Sedatives, Analgesics, and Paralytics

52. What are the most common side effects of the drug referred to in question 49?

_____

_____

_____

53. Which nondepolarizing NMBA has the longest duration of action?

_____

54. Which nondepolarizing NMBAs are used for intermediate duration?

_____

_____

_____

55. What type of patient could experience prolonged paralysis after discontinuation of pancuronium? Why?

_____

_____

_____

_____

56. Seizures have been associated with which nondepolarizing NMBA?

_____

57. Mast cell degranulation and histamine release, which may lead to peripheral vasodilation and hypotension, are associated with which nondepolarizing NMBA?

_____

58. Which nondepolarizing NMBAs are ideal for patients with renal and hepatic insufficiency?

_____

59. The nondepolarizing NMBA of choice for patients who are hemodynamically unstable, have cardiac disease, or are at risk of histamine release is:

_____

60. Give two side effects of the long-term use of neuromuscular blocking agents.

a. _____

b. _____

CRITICAL THINKING QUESTIONS

1. When a neuromuscular blocking agent is administered to a patient receiving ventilatory care, what ventilator alarms should be activated?

_____

_____

_____

2. Which type of opioid is best suited to a patient who has asthma? Why?

_____

_____

_____

CASE STUDY

The respiratory therapist checks on an ICU patient receiving ventilatory support with VC-SIMV. The ventilator settings are as follows: rate = 6 breaths/min, V_T = 600 mL, F_IO_2 = 0.4, PEEP = 5 cm H_2O. The mode was changed to VC-SIMV 1 hour ago because of asynchrony. The patient's legs are hanging over the bed railing, and his hands are on the ventilator tubing. The high pressure alarm is activating with every breath at a rate of 35 breaths/min. The patient is anxious and uncooperative and remains asynchronous with the ventilator.

1. What would be the most appropriate type of medication to deliver at this time?

_____

2. What concerns should the respiratory therapist have about the patient's ventilator settings?

_____

_____

_____

_____

NBRC-STYLE QUESTIONS

1. Which of the following drugs can be used to reverse the effects of benzodiazepines?
   a. Pseudocholinesterase
   b. Flumazenil (Romazicon)
   c. Fentanyl citrate (Sublimaze)
   d. Naloxone hydrochloride (Narcan)

2. The respiratory therapist is called to the postanesthesia care unit to assist in the weaning of a postoperative patient who had a cholecystectomy. The patient is 3 hours postop and is still apneic and receiving full ventilatory support. The medication(s) that could be used to facilitate ventilator weaning is (are) which of the following?
   1. Naloxone (Narcan)
   2. Propofol (Diprivan)
   3. Midazolam (Versed)
   4. Flumazenil (Romazicon)
   a. 1 and 4
   b. 2 and 4
   c. 1 and 3
   d. 2 and 3

3. An adult patient is in pain, panicky, and fighting the ventilator. The most appropriate medication to control this patient during mechanical ventilation is which of the following?
   a. Propofol (Diprivan)
   b. Haloperidol (Haldol)
   c. Fentanyl (Sublimaze)
   d. Succinylcholine (Anectine)

4. Which of the following is a fast-acting neuromuscular blocking agent that is often used to facilitate intubation?
   a. Vecuronium (Norcuron)
   b. Pancuronium (Pavulon)
   c. Midazolam (Versed)
   d. Succinylcholine (Anectine)

5. A mechanically ventilated patient who is hemodynamically unstable needs to be placed on pressure-controlled inverse ratio ventilation and will require paralysis. The most appropriate drug combination for this patient is which of the following?
   a. Succinylcholine (Anectine) and morphine
   b. Propofol (Diprivan) and fentanyl (Sublimaze)
   c. Atracurium (Tracrium) and midazolam (Versed)
   d. Cisatracurium (Nimbex) and flumazenil (Romazicon)

6. A patient with which of the following Ramsay scores is most likely to wean successfully from mechanical ventilation?
   a. 1
   b. 2
   c. 4
   d. 6

7. The depth of paralysis during neuromuscular blockade may be assessed with which of the following?
   a. Ramsay Scale
   b. Serum GABA levels
   c. TOF monitoring
   d. Level of sedation assessment

8. The neuromuscular blocking agent that causes histamine release is which of the following?
   a. Atracurium
   b. Cisatracurium
   c. Vecuronium
   d. Pancuronium

9. The neuromuscular blocking agent most appropriate for facilitating emergency intubation is which of the following?
   a. Pancuronium (Pavulon)
   b. Vecuronium (Norcuron)
   c. Atracurium (Tracrium)
   d. Succinylcholine (Anectine)

10. The neuromuscular blocking agent that can be used in patients with renal or hepatic insufficiency without producing prolonged paralysis is which of the following?
    a. Cisatracurium (Nimbex)
    b. Vecuronium (Norcuron)
    c. Pancuronium (Pavulon)
    d. Succinylcholine (Anectine)

16 Extrapulmonary Effects of Mechanical Ventilation

LEARNING OBJECTIVES

Upon completion of this chapter the reader will be able to do the following:

1. Explain the effects of positive pressure ventilation (PPV) on cardiac output and venous return to the heart.
2. Discuss the three factors that can influence cardiac output during positive pressure ventilation.
3. Explain the effects of positive pressure ventilation on gas distribution and pulmonary blood flow in the lungs.
4. Describe how positive pressure ventilation increases intracranial pressure (ICP).
5. Summarize the effects of positive pressure ventilation on renal and endocrine function.
6. Describe the effects of abnormal arterial blood gases (ABGs) on renal function.
7. Name five ways of assessing a patient's nutritional status.
8. Describe techniques that can be used to reduce some of the complications associated with mechanical ventilation.

KEY TERMS CROSSWORD PUZZLE

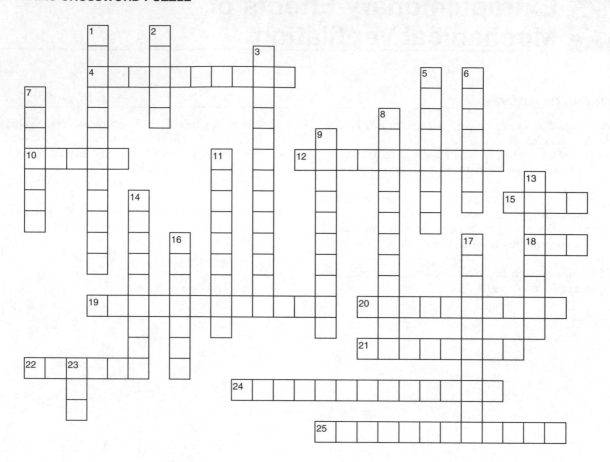

Across

4 This pressure is increased by an inflation hold (two words).
10 Gas always follows the path of _____ resistance.
12 Spontaneous inspiration increases blood flow to this structure (two words).
15 18 across plus ICP equals this (abbreviation).
18 The amount of blood flowing to the brain is determined by this (abbreviation).
19 A reduction in this decreases preload to the heart (two words).
20 Through the wall of an organ
21 Antidiuretic hormone release results in this.
22 The volume pumped out of a ventricle with one beat
24 This maneuver will increase inspiratory time (two words).
25 Inflammation of many nerves simultaneously

Down

1 A mechanism that maintains blood pressure (BP) in normal individuals receiving PPV
2 A function that can be altered by mechanical ventilation
3 This decreases with the use of PPV (two words).
5 Reduction in perfusion to an organ
6 The structural and functional unit of the kidney
7 Reductions in 19 across decrease this.
8 The pressure that falls with spontaneous inspiration
9 A drug used to avoid gastrointestinal bleeding
11 When an alveolus is overfilled, this capillary becomes thin.
13 A reflex that is blocked by 25 across
14 Compression of the heart
16 The vein that is visible when central venous pressure (CVP) is elevated
17 Urinary output will decrease when this capillary pressure decreases below 75 mm Hg.
23 Measuring this provides information about a patient's daily caloric requirements (abbreviation).

1. List the five bodily functions that positive pressure ventilation can significantly alter.

   a. _____   d. _____

   b. _____   e. _____

   c. _____

2. The physiologic effects of positive pressure ventilation on the cardiovascular system depend on what two factors?

   _____

3. Explain how spontaneous inspiration facilitates venous return to the right heart.

   _____

   _____

   _____

4. During what part of a spontaneous breath is right ventricular preload increased? Why?

   _____

   _____

5. During what part of a spontaneous breath is left ventricular preload decreased? Why?

   _____

   _____

   _____

6. An increase in central venous pressure will do what to the pressure gradient between systemic veins and the right heart?

   _____

Questions 7 through 9 refer to the following figure.

Point Y1
Pressure = 1 cm H_2O

Point Y2
Pressure = 3 cm H_2O

Point Y3
Pressure = 4.5 cm H_2O

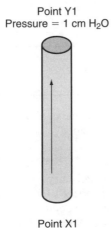 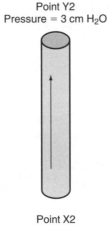 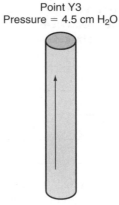

Point X1
Pressure = 5 cm H_2O

Point X2
Pressure = 5 cm H_2O

Point X3
Pressure = 5 cm H_2O

A   B   C

7. Which diagram represents the largest pressure gradient? _____

8. Which diagram represents the smallest pressure gradient? _____

Chapter **16** **Extrapulmonary Effects of Mechanical Ventilation**

9. If each tube in the figure represented the inferior vena cava, the "X" points represented systemic pressure, and the "Y" points represented central venous pressure, which diagram would have the most venous return?

_____

10. What effect does alveolar overdistention have on the pulmonary capillaries and right ventricular afterload?

_____

_____

_____

_____

_____

11. What conditions need to exist for the interventricular septum to move to the left during PPV?

_____

_____

12. How can PPV cause myocardial ischemia?

_____

_____

_____

_____

_____

_____

13. List the compensatory mechanisms responsible for the maintenance of systemic blood pressure during the ventilation of normal individuals:

_____

_____

_____

_____

14. What factors can block the body's compensatory mechanisms for maintaining arterial blood pressure while a patient is receiving PPV?

_____

_____

15. How can a respiratory therapist ensure that normal vascular reflexes are intact when PPV is being initiated?

_____

16. Normovolemic patients may experience decreases in cardiac output when positive end-expiratory pressure (PEEP) levels of _____ are used.

17. What three factors can influence cardiac output during PPV?

_____

_____

_____

18. How does PPV benefit the cardiac function of a patient with left ventricular dysfunction?

_____

_____

19. What pressure exerts the most influence on the extent of harmful effects caused by PPV?

_____

20. Calculate the mean airway pressure using the following parameters: peak inspiratory pressure (PIP) is 25 cm H_2O, T_I is 1 second, and respiratory rate is 12 breaths/minute.

_____

_____

_____

21. Add a 1-second inspiratory hold to the previous parameters and calculate the mean airway pressure.

_____

_____

_____

22. What happens to the mean airway pressure when an inspiratory hold is added?

_____

23. Calculate the mean airway pressure using the following parameters: PIP is 35 cm H_2O, PEEP is 10 cm H_2O, T_I is 1 second, and respiratory rate is 12 breaths/minute. (Notice the ΔP is the same as the PIP in the previous examples)

_____

_____

_____

_____

24. Calculate the mean airway pressure using the same parameters as in the previous example but add a 1-second inspiratory hold.

_____

_____

_____

25. What type of inspiratory flow produces uneven ventilation?

_____

26. The I:E ratios that are least likely to cause air trapping and significant hemodynamic complications are:

_____

27. What type of T_E allows for better alveolar emptying and less chance of developing auto-PEEP?

_____

28. The amount of mean airway pressure required to achieve a certain level of oxygenation may indicate:

_____

29. List five factors that influence mean airway pressure during mechanical ventilation:

a. _____

b. _____

c. _____

d. _____

e. _____

30. Explain why rapid inspiratory flow rates may produce lower mean airway pressures in patients with normal conducting airways.

_____

_____

31. For PEEP levels to affect cardiac output, what circumstances have to exist?

_____

_____

_____

32. In what circumstance would high levels of PEEP **not** cause a decrease in cardiac output?

_____

_____

_____

33. What is the cerebral perfusion pressure (CPP) when the intracranial pressure (ICP) is $18 cm H_2O$ and the mean systemic arterial blood pressure (MABP) is $85 cm H_2O$?

_____

34. How does PPV increase ICP?

_____

_____

_____

_____

35. How can an increased ICP be observed clinically?

_____

36. What effect does hyperventilation have on cerebral vessels?

_____

37. In what three ways is renal function altered by PPV?

a. _____

b. _____

c. _____

38. At what glomerular capillary pressure will urinary output become severely reduced?

_____

_____

39. What happens to kidney function when blood flow to the outer cortex decreases and flow to the inner cortex and outer medullary tissue increases?

_____

_____

40. Name the three hormones that are involved in fluid and electrolyte balance during PPV.

a. _____

b. _____

c. _____

41. PPV has what effects on each of these three hormones?

a. _____

b. _____

c. _____

42. Describe the effects of abnormal arterial blood gases on renal function.

_____

_____

43. What effects does PPV have on the pharmokinetics of certain drugs?

_____

_____

_____

44. How do PPV and PEEP affect the liver?

_____

_____

_____

_____

_____

45. What causes gastric distention in patients receiving PPV and how can it be reduced?

_____

_____

_____

46. Why are medical and surgical patients subject to malnutrition during serious illness?

_____

_____

_____

47. Name three deleterious effects that nutritional depletion can have on mechanically ventilated patients:

a. _____

b. _____

c. _____

48. Overfeeding can have what effects on a mechanically ventilated patient?

_____

_____

_____

49. Name five ways of assessing a patient's nutritional status:

a. _____

b. _____

c. _____

d. _____

e. _____

50. How can some of the complications associated with mechanical ventilation be reduced?

_____

_____

_____

CRITICAL THINKING QUESTIONS

1. Describe the cardiovascular effects, represented by the lettered arrows, that positive pressure ventilation is having on the heart in Figure 16-2.

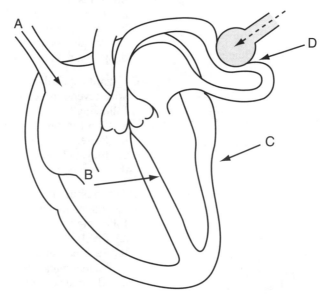

A. _____

_____

B. _____

_____

C. _____

_____

D. _____

_____

CASE STUDY

A 30-year-old, 5 ft 8 in, male postoperative patient with no lung disease is in the surgical intensive care unit receiving full mechanical support with the following ventilator settings: volume-controlled continuous mandatory ventilation (VC-CMV), rate 12, V_T 560 mL, flow rate 84 L/min, PEEP +10 cm H_2O, F_IO_2 50%. His peak inspiratory pressure is averaging around 30 cm H_2O and the plateau pressure is measured at 23 cm H_2O.

1) Calculate this patient's mean airway pressure.

_____

_____

_____

_____

_____

_____

Chapter **16**   **Extrapulmonary Effects of Mechanical Ventilation**

2) Analyze the patient's arterial blood gas on these ventilator settings: pH 7.38, PCO_2 42 mm Hg, PO_2 78 mm Hg, SaO_2 90%, HCO_3^- 23 mEq/L.

_____

_____

3) What is the most appropriate ventilator change at this time and why?

_____

_____

_____

_____

_____

NBRC-STYLE QUESTIONS

1. What effect does the normal thoracic pump mechanism have on cardiac output (CO)?
   a. Reduces CO in normal individuals
   b. Improves CO in healthy individuals
   c. Improves CO in individuals with disease
   d. Improves CO in mechanically ventilated patients only

2. During PPV and PPV with PEEP, which of the following is true regarding the thoracic pump mechanism?
   a. CO is decreased and venous return is decreased.
   b. Left ventricular output is decreased and CO is increased.
   c. Left ventricular stroke volume is decreased and CO is decreased.
   d. Right heart venous return is increased and blood pressure is increased.

3. The greatest reductions in venous return and cardiac output are most likely to occur during the use of which of the following ventilator modes?
   a. $CPAP = 8 \, cm \, H_2O$
   b. SIMV=10, V_T 450 mL
   c. CMV=12 with V_T 475 mL
   d. CMV=10, V_T 435 mL, PEEP +6 cm H_2O

4. A patient's inability to compensate for a diminished cardiac output during PPV will result in which of the following?
   a. Severe hemorrhaging
   b. Increased blood pressure
   c. Compromised perfusion
   d. Maintenance of normal blood pressure

5. For which of the following reasons are patients with ARDS less likely to experience hemodynamic changes during PPV, even with high ventilatory pressures?
   a. They have elevated systemic blood pressure.
   b. Their blood vessel walls have become too thick.
   c. Pressure is not transmitted to the pleural space.
   d. Pressure is lost in the poorly conductive airways.

6. Hazardous cardiovascular side effects in patients with severe bronchospasm are due to which of the following?
   a. Short inspiratory times
   b. Presence of auto-PEEP
   c. Elevated mean airway pressure
   d. Elevated peak inspiratory pressure

7. The pressure that has the most influence on the hemodynamic effects of PPV is which of the following?
   a. PEEP
   b. Peak pressure
   c. Plateau pressure
   d. Mean airway pressure

8. Methods of increasing mean airway pressure include which of the following?
   1. Increasing PEEP
   2. Increasing total cycle time
   3. Decreasing inspiratory time
   4. Adding an inflation hold
   a. 1 and 2 only
   b. 1 and 4 only
   c. 2 and 3 only
   d. 2 and 4 only

9. The risk of cardiovascular complications is least with the use of which of the following ventilator modes?
   a. PC-CMV
   b. VC-CMV with PEEP
   c. PC-SIMV with PS
   d. CPAP with PS

10. The anticipated effects of PPV on the kidneys include which of the following?
    1. Diuresis
    2. Sodium retention
    3. Decreased urinary output
    4. Increased creatinine excretion
    a. 1 and 2 only
    b. 2 and 3 only
    c. 3 and 4 only
    d. 1 and 4 only

17 Effects of Positive Pressure Ventilation on the Pulmonary System

LEARNING OBJECTIVES

Upon completion of this chapter, the reader will be able to do the following:

1. Recognize barotrauma or extra-alveolar air based on patient assessment.
2. Recommend appropriate action in patients with barotrauma.
3. Evaluate findings from a patient with acute respiratory distress syndrome (ARDS) to establish an optimum positive end-expiratory pressure (PEEP) and ventilation strategy.
4. Identify situations where chest wall rigidity can alter transpulmonary pressures and acceptable plateau pressures.
5. Name the types of ventilator-induced lung injury (VILI) caused by opening and closing of alveoli and overdistention of alveoli.
6. Compare the clinical findings in hyperventilation and hypoventilation.
7. Recommend ventilator settings in patients with hyperventilation and hypoventilation.
8. Identify a patient with air trapping.
9. Provide strategies to reduce auto-PEEP.
10. Suggest methods to reduce the work of breathing (WOB) during mechanical ventilation.
11. List the possible responses to an increase in mean airway pressure in a ventilated patient.
12. Describe the effects of positive pressure ventilation on pulmonary gas distribution and pulmonary perfusion in relation to normal spontaneous breathing.

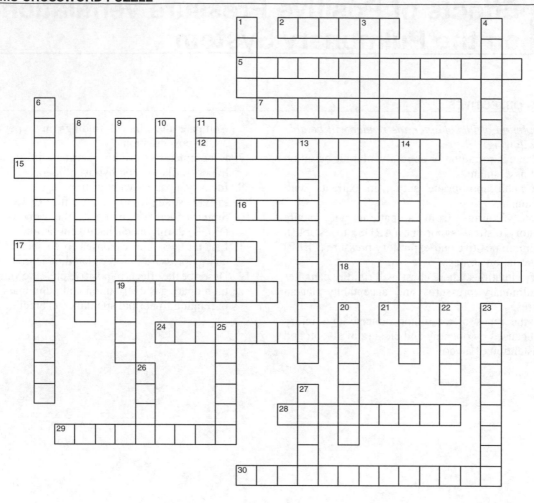

Across

2 Their presence increases risk of rupture of the lung.
5 Caused by too much volume in the alveoli
7 Caused by high levels of volume
12 General name for mediators released as a result of lung injury
15 Asynchrony caused by more than one breath type delivered by the ventilator
16 Abbreviation for lung injury at the level of the acinus
17 Caused by shear stress injury and loss of surfactant
18 Circulation of mediators causes this type of failure
19 Maneuver that causes pleural pressure to be positive
21 Asynchrony caused by inappropriate baseline settings
24 Caused by high levels of pressure
28 One type of mediator released as a result of lung injury
29 Touching subcutaneous emphysema feels like this.
30 Closing of lung units

Down

1 Asynchrony caused by inadequate gas speed
3 Atelectasis caused by high oxygen concentration
4 Asynchrony caused by dual control modes of ventilation (two words)
6 Inadequate alveolar ventilation
8 The sign indicative of a tension pneumothorax on chest radiograph
9 Type of hyperinflation caused by failure of lung volume to return to passive functional residual capacity (FRC)
10 Asynchrony caused by inappropriate sensitivity settings
11 Caused by release of inflammatory mediators from the lungs
13 A pneumothorax causes this to shift.
14 Opening of lung units
19 Abbreviation for lung injury as a consequence of mechanical ventilation
20 Asynchrony may cause this type of chest-abdominal movement.
22 Vascular area that hemorrhages due to alveolar trauma
23 This area of the lungs receives most blood flow in the supine position.
25 Another name for auto-PEEP or intrinsic PEEP
26 Abbreviation for diaphragm's electrical activity
27 Asynchrony caused by a very long inspiratory time

CHAPTER REVIEW QUESTIONS

1. Define *volutrauma*, *biotrauma*, and *atelectrauma*.

   _____

   _____

   _____

   _____

2. Briefly describe the difference between ventilator-induced lung injury (VILI) and ventilator-associated lung injury (VALI).

   _____

   _____

   _____

   _____

3. List five conditions that predispose a patient to barotrauma while he or she is being mechanically ventilated.

   a. _____

   b. _____

   c. _____

   d. _____

   e. _____

4. During patient ventilator system checks the respiratory therapist notes that one side of the patient's neck and face appear puffy. These areas feel crepitant to the touch. What is the most likely cause of this problem?

   _____

5. Rapid onset of increased peak airway pressures and decreasing lung compliance may be caused by

   _____.

6. What is the treatment for a tension pneumothorax?

   _____

   _____

   _____

7. A mechanically ventilated patient has developed a tension pneumothorax. How should the patient be ventilated until the appropriate treatment can begin?

   _____

   _____

8. List four clinical signs of a tension pneumothorax.

   a. _____

   b. _____

   c. _____

   d. _____

   e. _____

9. How would a chest radiograph of a patient with a tension pneumothorax look?

   _____

   _____

   _____

   _____

10. Air dissecting into the retroperitoneal space is known

    as: _____

11. What is the minimum transpulmonary pressure that has been associated with lung injury in animals?

    _____

12. List three examples of situations where lung injury may occur from abnormally high transpulmonary pressure.

    a. _____

    b. _____

    c. _____

13. Describe how volutrauma occurs.

    _____

    _____

    _____

    _____

    _____

14. In the clinical setting, how can chest wall movement be minimized to decrease the risk of lung injury from volutrauma?

    _____

    _____

15. What clinical situation puts a ventilated patient at risk of atelectrauma?

    _____

    _____

16. Name the types of ventilator-induced lung injury that are caused by opening and closing of alveoli and overdistention of alveoli.

_____

_____

17. Name two chemical mediators that are released when the alveolar epithelial cells are overstretched.

a. _____

b. _____

18. Describe how multiple organ dysfunction syndrome develops from overdistention of alveoli.

_____

_____

_____

_____

19. How can multiple organ dysfunction syndrome be avoided during mechanical ventilation?

_____

_____

_____

20. In what areas of the lung are ventilation and perfusion best matched during spontaneous ventilation in the supine position?

_____

_____

21. How are ventilation and perfusion altered during positive pressure ventilation (PPV) of a patient who is sedated and paralyzed?

_____

_____

_____

22. How can the changes in gas distribution during mechanical ventilation be minimized?

_____

23. How can positive pressure ventilation increase dead space?

_____

_____

_____

24. Why would the use of high volumes during PPV and PEEP cause an increase in pulmonary shunting?

_____

_____

_____

_____

25. How does mechanical ventilation cause increased pulmonary vascular resistance?

_____

_____

_____

26. Explain how hypoventilation can lead to cardiac dysrhythmias.

_____

27. What type of patient may benefit from permissive hypercapnia?

_____

28. List four reasons for patient-induced hyperventilation:

a. _____

b. _____

c. _____

d. _____

29. The cause of a right shift in the oxygen dissociation curve is: _____

30. Prolonged ventilator-induced hyperventilation can lead to what types of patient problems?

_____

_____

_____

31. What happens to the cerebrospinal fluid during prolonged hyperventilation with mechanical ventilation?

_____

_____

_____

32. When is the administration of intravenous bicarbonate indicated?

_____

_____

_____

_____

33. Why could administration of IV bicarbonate to a spontaneously breathing patient with a metabolic acidosis cause a problem?

_____

_____

_____

_____

34. List causes of metabolic alkalosis in the clinical

setting: _____

_____

_____

_____

35. What causes auto-PEEP without dynamic hyperinflation?

_____

_____

_____

_____

36. Ventilator-induced auto-PEEP can be created by:

_____

_____

_____

_____

37. What patient factors increase the risk of auto-PEEP?

_____

_____

_____

_____

38. On the graph below, draw a flow-time curve for volume-controlled continuous mandatory ventilation (VC-CMV), showing a "normal" exhalation and one exhibiting auto-PEEP.

_____

_____

39. What technique is used to detect the presence of auto-PEEP?

_____

_____

40. What patient and ventilator conditions must be present in order to detect auto-PEEP?

_____

_____

_____

41. How many time constants are necessary for the lungs to empty 98% of the inspired volume?

_____

_____

42. Define dynamic hyperinflation.

_____

_____

_____

43. What effects does the presence of auto-PEEP have on ventilator function?

_____

_____

_____

_____

Chapter **17** **Effects of PPV on the Pulmonary System**

44. Calculate static compliance for the following situation: $V_T = 525$ mL, PIP $= 43$ cmH_2O, $P_{plateau} = 30$ cmH_2O, set PEEP $= 12$ cmH_2O, auto-PEEP $= 5$ cmH_2O.

_____

_____

_____

_____

45. List four strategies that can be used to decrease auto-PEEP when the patient is receiving full ventilatory support:

a. _____

b. _____

c. _____

d. _____

46. List four modes of ventilation that may be used to decrease auto-PEEP in a patient who is intubated and has spontaneous breathing efforts:

a. _____

b. _____

c. _____

d. _____

47. When does pulmonary oxygen toxicity become a problem in adults and premature infants?

_____

_____

_____

48. If an F_1O_2 of greater than _____ is required, PEEP should be used. List four ways to assess pulmonary changes associated with oxygen toxicity.

a. _____

b. _____

c. _____

d. _____

49. What are the lower limit targets for oxygenation for patients receiving mechanical ventilation?

_____

50. The use of low tidal volumes with oxygen concentrations greater than 70% leads to:

_____

51. The normal inspiratory work of breathing is how much?

_____

52. Inspiratory work of breathing is considered high when it is greater than how much?

_____

53. A patient who has an increased work of breathing will most likely be experiencing what signs?

_____

54. Calculate the estimated work of breathing for a patient receiving mechanical ventilation with the following data: PIP $= 45$ cmH_2O, $P_{plateau} = 33$ cmH_2O, and $V_T = 475$ mL.

_____

_____

_____

_____

55. List four basic strategies for keeping the patient's WOB minimized.

a. _____

b. _____

c. _____

d. _____

56. List four signs of patient-ventilatory asynchrony.

a. _____

b. _____

c. _____

d. _____

57. Define trigger asynchrony and describe a method to avoid it.

_____

_____

_____

58. How does auto-PEEP cause trigger asynchrony?

_____

_____

_____

59. What should the initial flow be set at when using volume ventilation with a constant flow?

_____

_____

60. What type of breaths may provide more synchrony for a patient with high flow demands and why?

_____

_____

_____

61. What adjustment can be made during pressure-targeted ventilation to lessen the rapid rise of flow when a breath begins?

_____

_____

_____

62. What is cycle asynchrony and under what conditions can it occur?

_____

_____

_____

63. What strategies may be used to eliminate cycle asynchrony during mechanical ventilation with full support and spontaneous ventilation?

_____

_____

_____

64. What mode of ventilation delivers varying breath types which may result in mode asynchrony?

_____

_____

_____

65. When does PEEP asynchrony occur?

_____

_____

_____

66. How does closed-loop ventilation cause asynchrony?

_____

_____

_____

_____

_____

67. List at least five potential mechanical failures that can occur during mechanical ventilation.

a. _____

b. _____

c. _____

d. _____

e. _____

68. What seven complications can occur during mechanical ventilation?

a. _____

b. _____

c. _____

d. _____

e. _____

f. _____

g. _____

69. What hazards are associated with the use of both heat moisture exchangers (HMEs) and heated humidifiers?

_____

_____

_____

_____

70. What are the hazards associated with the use of HMEs?

_____

_____

_____

_____

Questions 1 and 2 refer to the figure below.

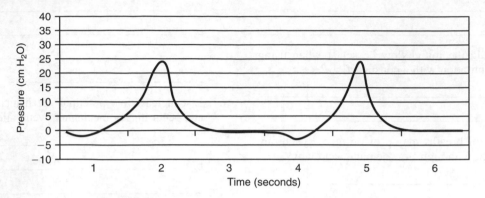

1. What problem is shown in this pressure-time curve?

_____

2. What change can be made to the ventilator settings to alleviate this problem?

_____

Questions 3 and 4 refer to the figure below.

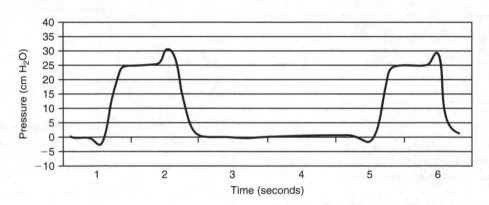

3. What problem is shown in this pressure-time curve?

_____

4. What change can be made to the ventilator settings to alleviate this problem?

_____

5. Which of the following patients will be more likely to develop auto-PEEP due to dynamic hyperinflation with a set rate of 12 breaths/minute? Why?

   Patient #1: airway resistance = $25\,cm\,H_2O/L/sec$ and static compliance = $50\,mL/cm\,H_2O$

   Patient #2: airway resistance = $6\,cm\,H_2O/L/sec$ and static compliance = $25\,mL/cm\,H_2O$

_____

_____

_____

_____

CASE STUDIES

Case Study 1

A patient who is 4 days post single-lung transplant is being mechanically ventilated. The remaining lung is fibrotic on chest x-ray and the transplanted lung is hyperinflated. The patient is unresponsive, cyanotic, and hypotensive. Her ideal body weight is 135 lb. She is being ventilated with VC-CMV and the flow sheet for the past few hours shows the following:

Time	Set Rate	Set V_T	Flow	PIP	F_IO_2	PEEP	pH	PCO_2	PO_2
0800	20	300	60	52	0.7	0	7.18	86	275
1000	22	300	60	50	1.0	0	7.15	94	504
1200	24	300	60	55	1.0	0	7.14	95	95
1400	40	320	60	60	1.0	0	7.06	110	125

$P_{plateau}$ at 1400 hours was 38 cm H_2O.

1. What is the most outstanding problem in this patient's ventilator course?

_____

_____

_____

2. What is the most likely cause of this problem?

_____

_____

_____

3. What complications is this patient at risk of developing?

_____

_____

_____

4. What should be the first change made to this patient's ventilator parameters?

_____

_____

_____

Case Study 2

A 65-year-old, 5 ft 10 in, male patient with chronic obstructive pulmonary disease (COPD) was intubated 3 days ago and is being mechanically ventilated with VC-CMV rate 14, $V_T = 550$ mL, $F_IO_2 = 30\%$, PEEP = +3 cm H_2O. This patient's baseline room air arterial blood gas is pH = 7.37, $PaCO_2 = 57$ mm Hg, $PaO_2 = 54$ mm Hg, $SaO_2 = 90\%$, $HCO_3^- = 30$ mEq/L. The arterial blood gases on the current ventilator setting are: pH 7.41, $PaCO_2$ 41 mm Hg, PaO_2 70 mm Hg, SaO_2 94%, and $HCO_3^- = 25$ mEq/L. The patient is placed on volume controlled-synchronized intermittent mandatory ventilation (VC-SIMV) to begin the weaning process and the mandatory rate is reduced to 6 breaths/min.

One hour after this change the respiratory therapist is called to the patient's room because the high respiratory rate alarm is sounding. The patient is diaphoretic, anxious, and tachycardic, and is using accessory muscles.

1. What is the most likely cause of this patient's failure to wean?

_____

_____

2. What could the respiratory therapist do to alleviate this problem?

_____

_____

_____

Chapter **17** **Effects of PPV on the Pulmonary System**

3. After 48 hours, the VC-SIMV is switched to pressure support ventilation (PSV) = 10 cm H_2O. The respiratory therapist observes the pressure-time scalar shown below. What is causing the spike at the end of the wave?

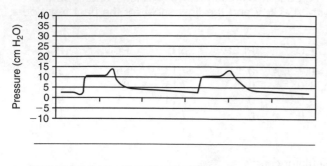

_____

_____

4. How can the problem be alleviated?

_____

NBRC-STYLE QUESTIONS

1. The major hazard(s) of oxygen therapy in association with mechanical ventilation include which of the following?
   1. Tachycardia
   2. Absorption atelectasis
   3. Oxygen-induced bradypnea
   4. Pulmonary oxygen toxicity
   a. 3 only
   b. 1 and 2 only
   c. 2 and 4 only
   d. 1, 3, and 4 only

2. Auto-PEEP should be suspected during which of the following observations?
   a. There is a prolonged postexpiratory pause.
   b. The patient coughs severely when suctioned.
   c. Expiration is continuous up to the next inspiration.
   d. The SIMV mandatory rate is set at 10 breaths/min.

3. The lung capacity that increases when auto-PEEP is present is which of the following?
   a. Vital capacity
   b. Inspiratory capacity
   c. Total lung capacity
   d. Functional residual capacity

4. Iatrogenic hyperventilation of a patient with a diagnosis of COPD may lead to which of the following consequences?
   1. Tetany
   2. Air trapping
   3. Cerebral edema
   4. Hypokalemia
   a. 2 only
   b. 1 and 3 only
   c. 2 and 4 only
   d. 1, 2, and 4 only

5. A patient who has been mechanically ventilated for 7 days has recently developed subcutaneous emphysema. Further assessment reveals cyanosis, signs of dyspnea, and a markedly elevated PIP. This patient is most likely experiencing which of the following?
   a. Pneumothorax
   b. Pneumoperitoneum
   c. Increased compliance
   d. Pneumomediastinum

6. The risk of volutrauma is increased for mechanically ventilated patients who exhibit which of the following?
   a. Increased P_{ta}
   b. Decreased P_{alv}
   c. Increased P_L
   d. Decreased P_{awo}

7. The amount of bicarbonate replacement given to a patient with severe metabolic acidosis who weighs 145 lb and has a base deficit of 10 should be which of the following?
   a. 55 mEq
   b. 110 mEq
   c. 220 mEq
   d. 242 mEq

8. Failure to recognize a patient's trigger efforts is known as which of the following?
   a. Mode asynchrony
   b. Flow asynchrony
   c. Trigger asynchrony
   d. Closed-loop ventilation asynchrony

9. An increase in a patient's assist rate followed by a rise in PIP and drop in exhaled tidal volume is most often associated with which of the following?
   a. Auto-PEEP
   b. Mode asynchrony
   c. PEEP asynchrony
   d. Subcutaneous emphysema

10. The presence of fine, late inspiratory crackles may lead to which of the following lung injuries?
    1. Biotrauma
    2. Shear stress
    3. Surfactant alteration
    4. Subcutaneous emphysema
    a. 1 and 2 only
    b. 2 and 3 only
    c. 1 and 4 only
    d. 3 and 4 only

Chapter 17 Effects of PPV on the Pulmonary System

18 Problem Solving and Troubleshooting

LEARNING OBJECTIVES

Upon completion of this chapter, the reader will be able to do the following:

1. Identify various types of technical problems encountered during mechanical ventilation of critically ill patients and describe the steps that can be used to protect a patient when problems occur.
2. Name at least two possible causes for each of the following alarm situations: low pressure alarm, high pressure alarm, low PEEP/CPAP alarms, apnea alarm, low or high tidal volume alarm, low or high minute volume alarm, low or high respiratory rate alarm, low or high F_IO_2 alarm, low source gas pressure or power input alarm, ventilator inoperative alarm, and technical error message.
3. Determine the cause of a problem using a graphic from a patient-ventilator system.
4. Assess a description of a patient situation and recommend a solution.
5. Describe the signs and symptoms associated with patient-ventilator asynchrony.
6. Explain the correct procedure for determining whether a problem originates with the patient or with the ventilator in patient-ventilator asynchrony.
7. List four ways the addition of a nebulizer powered by an external source gas can affect ventilator function.
8. Recognize abnormalities in ventilator graphics and patient response in the event of inadequate gas flow delivery to a patient.
9. Identify the causes and potential problems related to electrolyte imbalances.
10. Recognize the signs and symptoms of a respiratory infection.
11. Identify a problem associated with an artificial airway or a mask used for noninvasive positive pressure ventilation.
12. Recognize the presence of auto-PEEP using ventilator graphics.
13. Suggest appropriate interventions for a patient who has experienced a right mainstem intubation and for a patient with a pneumothorax, using physical assessment data.
14. Describe potential problems associated with using a heated humidification system during mechanical ventilation.
15. Use a ventilator flow-volume loop to assess a patient's response to bronchodilator therapy.
16. Make recommendations about ventilator parameters for a patient with acute respiratory distress syndrome.
17. Recommend adjustment of flow-cycle criteria during pressure support ventilation based on ventilator graphics.

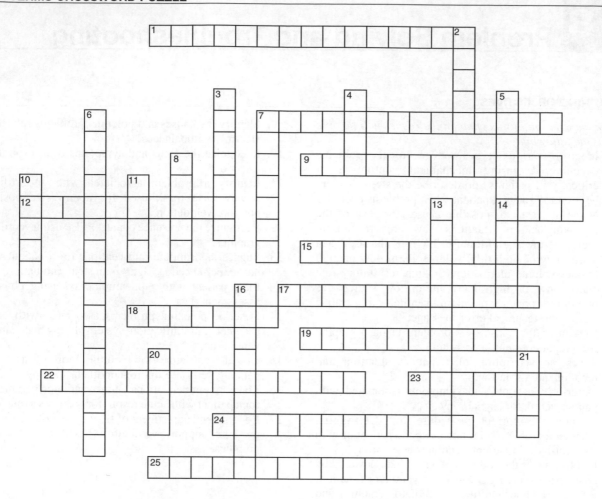

Across

1 The type of interference caused by a cell phone
7 Fluid in the lungs (two words)
9 A life-threatening cause of severe patient distress
12 The artery that may rupture within 3 weeks after a tracheostomy
14 Continuous suction endotracheal tube (abbreviation)
15 An indicator of severe cardiopulmonary distress
17 Out of synchrony with the ventilator
18 Waveform _____ is caused by oscillation of air in the patient-ventilator circuit at the beginning of inspiration.
19 Without synchrony
22 Identification and resolution of technical malfunctions in the patient-ventilator system
23 Abnormal accumulation of edematous fluid within the peritoneal cavity
24 Smooth muscle contraction in the lungs
25 A type of therapy that breaks up blood clots

Down

2 Active exhalation during pressure support ventilation is a common cause of this type of asynchrony.
3 An uncomfortable situation
4 This type of asynchrony occurs when more than one breath type is delivered.
5 Inward protrusion of intercostal spaces
6 Blood clot in the lungs (two words)
7 The person attached to the ventilator
8 Alert for a clinician
10 The endotracheal tube (ET) will slip into this bronchus.
11 An unintentional bend in the endotracheal tube
13 Especially profuse perspiration
16 Radiograph of blood vessels
20 The type of asynchrony that occurs when gas speed is inadequate
21 A patient disconnect will cause this.

CHAPTER REVIEW QUESTIONS

1. Define the term *problem*.

   _____

   _____

2. Define *troubleshooting* in the context of mechanical ventilation.

   _____

   _____

   _____

3. When responding to an activated ventilator alarm, what is the respiratory therapist's first priority?

   _____

   _____

4. To establish the respiratory therapist's first priority, what assessments must be made?

   _____

   _____

   _____

5. If a serious ventilatory problem is detected, what should the respiratory therapist's next step be?

   _____

   _____

6. What are the advantages and disadvantages of manually ventilating a patient when a problem is detected?

   _____

   _____

   _____

   _____

   _____

7. List the physical signs of distress that a patient receiving mechanical ventilation might exhibit.

   _____

   _____

   _____

8. What equipment, techniques, or data can be used to help identify the cause of a patient's sudden distress while being mechanically ventilated?

   _____

   _____

   _____

9. List six patient-related causes of sudden respiratory distress that originate within the patient's lungs.

   a. _____

   b. _____

   c. _____

   d. _____

   e. _____

   f. _____

10. List six nonpulmonary patient-related causes of sudden respiratory distress.

    a. _____

    b. _____

    c. _____

    d. _____

    e. _____

    f. _____

11. List the six types of patient-ventilator asynchrony that can cause sudden respiratory distress.

    a. _____

    b. _____

    c. _____

    d. _____

    e. _____

    f. _____

12. Aside from patient-ventilator asynchrony, what ventilator-related issues can cause sudden respiratory distress in patients?

    _____

    _____

13. How can the respiratory therapist distinguish the difference between severe distress caused by a ventilator-related or patient-related problem?

_____

_____

_____

14. Describe the seven steps needed to manage sudden severe distress in a ventilator-supported patient.

a. _____

b. _____

c. _____

d. _____

e. _____

f. _____

g. _____

15. An oral ET should be approximately at what mark for men and for women? What are the appropriate ranges for each?

_____

_____

16. What steps should be taken if a suction catheter cannot be passed down the ET of a patient in severe respiratory distress (patient is not biting the tube)?

_____

_____

17. What clinical manifestation should a respiratory therapist look for when a tension pneumothorax is suspected during positive pressure ventilation?

_____

_____

18. If a tension pneumothorax is strongly suspected and cardiopulmonary arrest is imminent, what action should be taken?

_____

_____

19. What signs suggest that a patient is experiencing bronchospasm while receiving mechanical ventilation?

_____

_____

_____

20. What other patient problems can cause wheezing?

_____

21. How can problems due to secretions be minimized during mechanical ventilation?

_____

_____

22. What is the difference in onset between cardiogenic and noncardiogenic pulmonary edema?

_____

_____

_____

23. How does auto-PEEP affect the flow-time scalar and the flow-volume loop?

_____

_____

24. List conditions that may stimulate the respiratory center output.

_____

_____

25. Describe how the presence of abdominal distention can cause atelectasis, ventilation/perfusion abnormalities, and hypoxemia?

_____

_____

_____

26. The rapid onset of hypoxemia, tachycardia, tachypnea, and hypertension, along with a decrease in end-tidal CO_2, is indicative of what type of patient problem? How can this problem be confirmed and treated?

_____

_____

_____

27. What are the common sites for leaks to occur in the patient-ventilator system?

_____

_____

_____

28. How is a manual leak test performed on a ventilator connected to a patient?

_____

_____

_____

29. List six causes of trigger asynchrony.

a. _____

b. _____

c. _____

d. _____

e. _____

f. _____

30. List at least four common causes of a low-pressure alarm situation.

a. _____

b. _____

c. _____

d. _____

31. List nine common causes of a high-pressure alarm situation.

a. _____

b. _____

c. _____

d. _____

e. _____

f. _____

g. _____

h. _____

i. _____

32. If the peak inspiratory pressure (PIP) is 30 cm H_2O, what should the low- and high-pressure alarms be set at?

_____

_____

33. Name two conditions that would trigger a low PEEP/CPAP alarm.

a. _____

b. _____

34. List five potential causes for triggering an apnea alarm.

a. _____

b. _____

c. _____

d. _____

e. _____

35. List two potential causes for triggering a low-source gas pressure alarm.

a. _____

b. _____

36. Name two potential causes for a power-input alarm.

a. _____

b. _____

37. What is the most likely cause of a "ventilator inoperative" alarm?

_____

_____

38. Describe the alarm situations and ventilator graphics that a leak in the patient-ventilator system would cause.

_____

_____

_____

_____

39. What types of graphics will allow the respiratory therapist to detect inadequate flow?

_____

_____

40. The phenomenon caused by the oscillation of air in the patient-ventilator circuit and at the upper airway at the beginning of inspiration is known as:

_____

41. What can be done to alleviate the problem caused by the phenomenon in the previous question?

_____

_____

42. Name three problems that may cause the expiratory portion of the volume-time curve to go below baseline.

a. _____

b. _____

c. _____

43. How does an externally powered nebulizer affect ventilator function?

_____

_____

_____

_____

44. A leak in the endotracheal tube cuff will cause which alarms to be activated?

_____

_____

45. Compare the findings from a right mainstem intubation and from a left and right tension pneumothorax by completing the chart below.

Clinical Findings	Right Mainstem Intubation	Left-sided Pneumothorax	Right-sided Pneumothorax
PIP			
$P_{plateau}$			
Breath sounds			
Chest movement			
Percussion			
Tracheal shift			

46. How can a pulmonary embolism be detected during mechanical ventilation?

_____

_____

_____

47. During mechanical ventilation with pressure controlled-continuous mandatory ventilation (PC-CMV), the low tidal volume alarm becomes activated on every breath; there is no leak in the system. What could be the cause of this alarm?

_____

_____

48. How can a respiratory therapist determine the cause of an increasing peak inspiratory pressure?

_____

_____

_____

_____

49. What type of asynchrony most commonly occurs during pressure support ventilation?

_____

_____

50. How can the asynchrony from the previous question be detected on ventilator graphics?

_____

_____

51. What type of problem would cause a high pressure alarm to become activated intermittently?

_____

_____

52. What type of problem should the respiratory therapist suspect when a ventilator patient exhibits sudden respiratory distress and a suction catheter cannot be passed through the endotracheal tube? What action should be taken?

_____

_____

_____

53. What steps can be taken to decrease auto-PEEP?

_____

_____

_____

54. What situations can cause the I:E ratio indicator and alarm to be activated?

_____

_____

55. A respiratory therapist responding to a ventilator alarm finds that the high respiratory rate alarm is activated. The ventilator is set to VC-CMV rate 12. What are some possible reasons for this activated alarm?

_____

_____

_____

CRITICAL THINKING QUESTIONS

Questions 1 through 4 refer to the following scenario.

You are the respiratory therapist who responds to a ringing ventilator alarm. The patient has been receiving mechanical ventilation for the past 3 days following an exacerbation of congestive heart failure and pneumonia. She has been unresponsive to verbal stimuli during this period. Her ventilator settings are volume controlled-continuous mandatory ventilation (VC-CMV), set rate 12 breaths/min, tidal volume 475 mL, F_IO_2 50%, and PEEP 5 cm H_2O. The PIP has been averaging 28 cm H_2O and the $P_{plateau}$ about 21 cm H_2O. As you approach the patient you note that the alarm panel indicates a high-pressure condition along with low exhaled tidal volume and low exhaled minute volume. The patient's high pressure alarm threshold is set at 40 cm H_2O and the returned volume is 175 mL.

1. What action should the respiratory therapist take at this time?

_____

_____

_____

_____

2. Name three conditions that could cause this situation.

a. _____

b. _____

c. _____

3. Describe the best course of action to remedy each of the three conditions mentioned in the previous answer.

_____

_____

_____

_____

4. Why are the low exhaled tidal volume and low exhaled minute volume active along with the high pressure alarm?

_____

_____

_____

_____

_____

Chapter **18**   **Problem Solving and Troubleshooting**

Questions 5 and 6 refer to the following scenario.

A patient recently weaned from full ventilatory support has just been switched to CPAP +10 cm H_2O with pressure support of 25 cm H_2O. After a few spontaneous breaths on the CPAP with pressure support, the patient developed respiratory distress. The patient does not seem to be able to trigger the pressure supported breaths and the ventilator's apnea alarm has been activated.

5. Explain two possible causes for this patient's respiratory distress.

   a. _____

   b. _____

6. What actions could correct these possible causes?

   _____

   _____

   _____

CASE STUDIES

Case Study 1

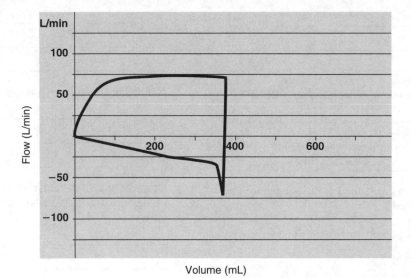

1. The flow-volume loop shown in the preceding figure is for a patient receiving mechanical ventilation. What type of problem is demonstrated in this flow-volume loop?

   _____

2. What can be done to solve this problem?

   _____

A 42-year-old male had surgery to repair a crushed hip and femur fractures that occurred in a motor vehicle accident. Five hours after surgery, the patient continues to receive positive pressure ventilation. Up to now the patient's condition has been stable, but he has been unconscious. At 1810 hours, a sudden change in the patient's vital signs has brought the respiratory therapist to the patient's bedside. The pulse oximetry reading has dropped from 96% to 87%, and BP has risen from 136/82 to 160/100 mm Hg. The table below shows the last patient-ventilator checks.

Date	5/29	5/29	5/29	5/29
Time	1400	1610	1750	1810
Mode	PC-CMV	PC-CMV	PC-CMV	PC-CMV
Set rate	12	12	12	12
Total rate	12	12	20	25
Volume	620 mL	628 mL	625 mL	615 mL
T_I	1 second	1 second	1 second	1 second
Waveform	square	square	square	square
PIP (cm H_2O)	30	28	32	33
$P_{plateau}$ (cm H_2O)	23	21	22	20
PEEP (cm H_2O)	5	5	5	↑ 8
F_IO_2	0.4	0.4	0.4	↑ 0.6
Breath sounds	bilateral clear	bilateral clear	bilateral clear	bilateral clear
BP (mm Hg)	136/82	132/80	155/88	160/100
HR (BPM)	96	94	125	128
SpO_2	96%	96%	96%	87%
$P_{ET}CO_2$ (mm Hg)	36	36	34	26
ABGs				
pH	7.43	—	—	7.47
$PaCO_2$ (mm Hg)	39	—	—	30
PaO_2 (mm Hg)	98	—	—	78

1. The patient is now in obvious respiratory distress. What action should the respiratory therapist take at this time?

_____

_____

2. Nothing that is done seems to relieve this patient's respiratory distress. What is the most likely cause of this problem?

_____

_____

A 62-year-old woman is receiving ventilatory support with volume ventilation. She had abdominal surgery 10 hours ago. She has no history of smoking. Over the past few hours, the following patient information was gathered:

Time	0700	0900	1000
Volume	450 mL	450 mL	450 mL
PIP	18 cm H_2O	24 cm H_2O	27 cm H_2O
$P_{plateau}$	13 cm H_2O	12 cm H_2O	14 cm H_2O

1. What is the most likely cause of the increase in PIP between 7 and 10 AM?

_____

_____

2. List some of the problems that can cause this type of increase in PIP.

_____

_____

3. What actions should the respiratory therapist take to determine the source of this patient's problem?

_____

_____

NBRC-STYLE QUESTIONS

1. During pressure control ventilation, the alarm that identifies worsening lung compliance is which of the following?
   a. Low PEEP/CPAP
   b. High respiratory rate
   c. Low V_{Texh}
   d. High PIP

2. Identify the problem in the following flow-time scalar.

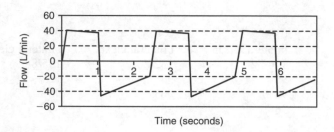

   a. Auto-PEEP
   b. Excessively prolonged T_E
   c. Inadequate T_I
   d. Increased airway resistance

3. The problem represented in the pressure-time scalar below may be solved by which of the following?

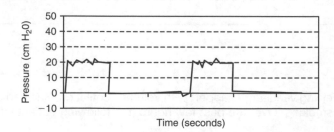

   a. Changing the flow waveform
   b. Increasing pressure sensitivity
   c. Increasing inspiratory rise time
   d. Increasing the peak pressure

4. The problem indicated in the flow-volume loop below is which of the following?

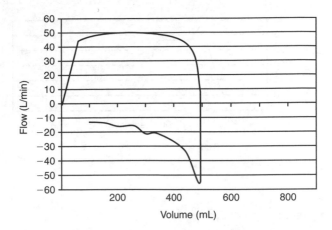

a. Increase in airway resistance
b. Active exhalation against inspiration
c. Leak in the patient-ventilator system
d. Auto-PEEP

5. The problem indicated in the pressure-volume loop below, obtained during VC-CMV, can be solved by which of the following?

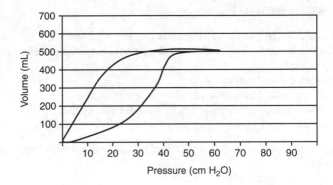

   1. Suctioning of the ET tube
   2. Switching to PC-CMV
   3. Lower the V_T in VC-CMV
   4. Administering a bronchodilator
a. 1 and 2
b. 2 and 3
c. 3 and 4
d. 1 and 4

6. The problem that could cause the pressure-time scalar below is which of the following?

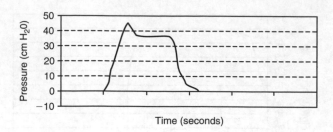

   1. Bronchoconstriction
   2. High airway resistance
   3. Alveolar overdistention
   4. Decreased lung compliance
   a. 1 and 2
   b. 2 and 3
   c. 3 and 4
   d. 1 and 4

7. The respiratory therapist is assessing a mechanically ventilated patient who has developed sudden respiratory distress. The respiratory therapist notes that the 15-mm ET adapter is at the level of the patient's teeth. The suspected airway problem is which of the following?
   a. Cuff rupture or leakage
   b. Rupture of the innominate artery
   c. Patient biting the ET tube
   d. The ET tube has slipped into the right mainstem bronchus.

8. The respiratory therapist is unable to pass a suction catheter into a patient's ET tube or to ventilate the patient manually with a resuscitator bag. Deflation of the cuff does not relieve the patient's distress. The most appropriate action is which of the following?
   a. Reinflate the cuff and attempt ventilation again.
   b. Remove the ET tube and provide bag-mask ventilation.
   c. Keep the cuff inflated and attempt ventilation again with 100% oxygen.
   d. Deflate the cuff, suction the upper airway, and provide bag-mask ventilation.

9. The respiratory therapist strongly suspects that the patient has a tension pneumothorax. What should the RT do in this life-threatening situation?
   a. Suction the patient's ET tube vigorously
   b. Insert a chest tube into the sixth intercostal space
   c. Insert a 14- or 16-gauge needle into the second intercostal space
   d. Remove the patient from the ventilator and provide resuscitation

10. While providing mechanical ventilatory support for a conscious patient, the respiratory therapist notes dyspnea, wheezing, and increased use of accessory muscles of breathing. These clinical findings are most closely associated with which of the following?
    a. Cuff leakage
    b. Bronchospasm
    c. Pneumothorax
    d. Increased secretions

11. What should the respiratory therapist check first when a low pressure alarm is activated on a ventilator?
    a. Apnea parameters
    b. Patient connection
    c. 50 psi gas source
    d. Ventilator electronics

12. What problem must be present to cause simultaneous activation of the low pressure, low volume, and low $\dot{V}_E$ alarms?
    a. Inadequate flow setting
    b. Ventilator asynchrony
    c. Patient-ventilator system leak
    d. Inappropriate trigger sensitivity

19 Basic Concepts of Noninvasive Positive Pressure Ventilation

LEARNING OBJECTIVES

Upon completion of this chapter, the reader will be able to do the following:

1. Define *noninvasive ventilation* and discuss the three basic noninvasive techniques.
2. Discuss the clinical and physiological benefits of noninvasive positive pressure ventilation (NIV).
3. Identify the selection and exclusion criteria for NIV application in the acute and chronic care settings.
4. Compare the types of ventilators used for noninvasive ventilation.
5. Explain the importance of humidification during NIV application.
6. Describe the factors that will influence the F_1O_2 from a portable pressure targeted ventilator.
7. Identify possible causes of rebreathing CO_2 during NIV administration from a portable pressure targeted ventilator.
8. Compare the advantages and disadvantages of the various types of interfaces for the application of NIV.
9. List the steps used in the initiation of NIV.
10. Discuss several factors that affect the delivery of aerosols during NIV.
11. Identify several indicators of success for patients on NIV.
12. Make recommendations for ventilator changes based on observation of the patient's respiratory status, acid-base status, or oxygenation status.
13. Recognize potential complications of NIV.
14. Provide optional solutions to complications of NIV.
15. Describe two basic approaches to weaning a patient from NIV.

Chapter **19** **Basic Concepts of Noninvasive Positive Pressure Ventilation**

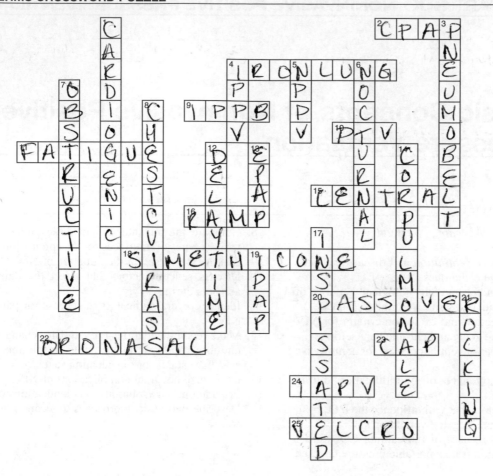

Across

2 First-choice therapy indicated to treat obstructive sleep apnea (OSA)

4 Type of ventilator used during the polio epidemic (two words)

9 Abbreviation for a therapy used to deliver periodic aerosolized medication with positive pressure breaths

10 Another name for bi-level continuous positive airway pressure (CPAP) ventilators (abbreviation)

11 A symptom of chronic hypoventilation

15 A type of apnea that originates in the brain

16 A setting that allows positive pressure levels to gradually increase

18 An anti-gas agent

20 A type of heated humidifier used to prevent or treat mucosal dehydration with NIV

22 A type of mask that covers both nose and mouth

23 Abbreviation for a type of pneumonia acquired outside the hospital

24 Abbreviation for abdominal displacement ventilator

25 The material that fastens the head gear.

Down

1 A type of pulmonary edema due to a weak heart

3 A type of abdominal displacement ventilator

4 Abbreviation for another name for positive pressure ventilation

5 Abbreviation for the use of positive pressure ventilation via a mask

6 A type of hypoventilation that occurs at night

7 Type of sleep apnea that occurs from the collapse of the upper airway during sleep

8 A portable negative pressure device (two words)

12 The setting that controls the amount of time it takes for the positive pressure level to gradually increase (two words)

13 The expiratory setting for bi-level CPAP (abbreviation)

14 Right heart failure due to an obstructive pulmonary disease (two words)

17 Secretions that are dried up are _____.

19 The inspiratory setting for bi-level CPAP (abbreviation)

21 A type of bed that is motorized and which moves continuously in a longitudinal plane

CHAPTER REVIEW QUESTIONS

1. Define *noninvasive ventilation*.

delivery of mech. vent w/o an endotrachial airway

2. What are the three basic methods of applying NIV?
   a. negative pressure vent.
   b. abdominal displacement vent.
   c. positive pressure vent.

3. How do negative pressure ventilators operate?

intermittently applying neg. pressure to entire body. Neg. press. is transmitted across the chest wall → pleural space → alveolar space. Exhalation is passive.

4. Name two negative pressure ventilators.
   a. iron lung
   b. chest curiass

5. What is the most significant benefit of NIV?

avoid invasive vent.

6. What is the primary goal of NIV in the acute-care setting?

avoid intubation

7. List at least six clinical benefits of NIV in the acute care setting.
   a. decrease need for intubation
   b. decrease nosocomial pneumonia
   c. ↓ length of ICU stay
   d. ↓ hospital stay
   e. ↓ mortality
   f. improve pt. comfort

8. List at least three clinical benefits of NIV in the chronic care setting.
   a. improve duration & quality of sleep
   b. improve functional capacity
   c. prolong survival

9. How does the use of NIV in acute respiratory failure improve gas exchange?

By resting the resp. muscles & ↑ alveolar ventilation

10. What are the benefits of using NIV via a facemask instead of invasive mechanical ventilation in the treatment of acute respiratory failure due to chronic obstructive pulmonary disease (COPD)?

Reduces need for intubation, ↓ duration of mechanical vent, decreases complications.

11. What are the benefits of using NIV for patients with status asthmaticus complicated by CO_2 retention?

improved gas exchange, ↓ CO_2, rapid improvement in vitals

12. When a patient with cardiogenic pulmonary edema does not respond to conventional pharmacologic and oxygen therapy, what types of NIV have been shown to be effective?

Mask CPAP

13. The clinical disorders that manifest in chronic respiratory failure which require NIV as supportive therapy include:

chronic hypoventilation, nocturnal desaturation, resp. muscle fatigue, poor sleep quality

14. List the five symptoms of chronic hypoventilation.
   a. fatigue
   b. morning headache
   c. daytime hypersomnolance
   d. cognitive dysfunction
   e. dyspnea
   f.

15. How many hours must a patient with chronic hypoventilation use NIV to achieve clinical benefits?

4 - 6 hrs.

Chapter **19** Basic Concepts of Noninvasive Positive Pressure Ventilation

16. The use of NIV only at night or intermittently during the day for patients with neuromuscular disorders shows what clinical benefits?

Daytime gas exchange & resp. muscle strength

17. What are the criteria for using NIV with patients who have chronic stable COPD?

If they have severe daytime CO_2 retention (>52) & nocturnal hypoventilation

18. What role does NIV play in the treatment of advanced cystic fibrosis?

Supports pt. while awaiting lung transplant

19. When an OSA patient continues to hypoventilate and to experience nocturnal desaturation while receiving CPAP, what therapy is indicated?

NIV

20. What are the benefits of reducing the number of days a patient is invasively ventilated?

↓ risk of infection, ↓ mortality rate & ↓ health care costs

21. What can NIV do for a patient who exhibits fatigue following extubation?

↓ WOB & maintain adequate gas exchange for pt. w/ fatigue

22. What role does NIV play in "end-of-life" situations?

provide relief from severe dyspnea, & preserve pt. comfort

23. List nine indications for the use of NIV for adult patients with acute respiratory failure.

a. acute exacerbation of COPD
b. acute asthma
c. hypoxemic resp. failure
d. CAP
e. cardiogenic pulm. edema
f. immunocomprimised pts.
g. post-op pts.
h. post extubation
i. do not intubate

24. What are the signs and symptoms of respiratory distress in patients who need ventilatory assistance?

tachypnea, use of acess. muscles, paradoxial breathing

25. What are the blood gas criteria for adult patients who need ventilatory support due to moderate to severe respiratory failure?

$CO_2 > 45$, $pH < 7.35$, or $O_2 < 200$

26. What are the exclusion criteria for NIV?

Resp. arrest or immediate intubation, inability to protect airway, excessive secretions, agitation/confusion, facial deformities, uncooperative

27. What is the final consideration in the selection of patients with acute respiratory failure for NIV?

Potential reversibility

28. What are the symptoms of nocturnal hypoventilation and poor sleep quality?

excessive fatigue, morning headache, daytime hypersomnalance, cog. dysfunction, dyspnea

29. What are the physiologic criteria for the institution of NIV in a chronic care setting for patients with restrictive thoracic disorders and neuromuscular disorders?

$CO_2 > 45$, Nocturnal desat, > 88 for longer than 5 MINS.

30. What are the physiologic criteria for the institution of NIV for patients with severe stable COPD in a chronic care setting?

$CO_2 > 55$, CO_2 50-54 for 5 consecutive mins W/ SaTs < 88%

31. The physiologic criteria for the institution of NIV for patients with nocturnal hypoventilation include:

PSG evidence of OSA, unresponsive to CPAP

32. How do portable pressure targeted ventilators maintain pressure levels and flush exhaled gases from the circuit?

Single-circuit gas delivery w/ an intentional mask port for pt. exhalation

33. What are the trigger, limit, and cycle variables for the bi-level CPAP ventilators?

flow & time triggered, pressure limited & flow & time cycled

34. What are the inspiratory and expiratory settings called on the bi-level CPAP ventilators?

IPAP & EPAP

35. The typical ranges for the inspiratory and expiratory settings on the bi-level CPAP ventilators are:

IPAP = 2-30, EPAP = 2-20

36. Most PTVs offer what modes of ventilatory support?

CPAP, PSV, S/T

37. What determines the patient's tidal volume during the use of a PTV?

gradient b/t IPAP & EPAP, inspiratory time, inspiratory effort

38. Where is the source for unintentional leaks in a PTV?

around their mask

39. What makes the PTVs able to flow trigger even though there are intentional and unintentional leaks in the system?

Flow

40. What two controls are incorporated in newer PTVs to improve synchronization between patient and ventilator?

a. inspiratory sensitivity
b. expiratory levels

41. What features are now incorporated in the newer PTVs to improve patient comfort?

Rise/RAMP, Delay

42. What are the four factors that cause the F_1O_2 for a portable PTV to be variable?

a. O_2 flow rate
b. type of leak
c. where O_2 is bled in
d. IPAP & EPAP

43. How can precise oxygen concentrations be delivered through a PTV?

O_2 blender

44. What effect will an inadequate continuous flow from a PTV have on the patient?

prevents exhaled gases to exit the system

45. The flow of gas through the leak port of a PTV is dependent on what settings?

EPAP & I:E ratio

46. How can CO_2 rebreathing be minimized with a PTV?

EPAP lvl of 4 or ↑

47. What advantages do the new-generation portable ventilators have over the original portable pressure targeted ventilator?

diff. modes, alarms & graphics

185

48. What are the advantages and disadvantages of using an adult acute care ventilator for NIV?

good for diff. modes, & alarms
bad b/c some try to compensate for leaks

49. When using an adult acute care ventilator for NIV, which mode will make the patient most comfortable and why?

PC-CMV b/c cycling to exhalation is a function of time instead of flow

50. Why is it important for heated humidity to be added during NIV?

reduces dryness

51. What type of heated humidifier is recommended for NIV? Why?

heated-passover

52. Which type of NIV/CPAP interface is most widely used?

nasal mask

53. What advantages does the nasal mask have over the full face mask during the administration of NIV?

easier to fit & secure
better pt. tolerated
allows clearing of secretions & coughing

54. The two most common disadvantages of the nasal mask are:

air leaks & skin irritations

55. What type of NIV interface should be used when a patient has large air leaks through the mouth?

oronasal or full-face

56. What are the major concerns about using the full face mask and total face mask for the administration of NIV?

risk of aspiration
asphyxia
↑ DS

57. How much dead space volume does a full face mask have?

250 ML

58. What are the advantages of using a mouthpiece or lip seal over a nasal mask?

no leaks, ↓ O₂ rebreathing

59. In what position should the patient be when NIV is being initiated?

sitting upright

60. When the NIV is turned on for the first time, what ventilator setting should be used?

EPAP 4-5, IPAP 8-10

61. After ensuring proper mask size and fit what steps should be taken to initiate NIV?

hold mask to pts. face to get used to it, then apply to face & secure straps

62. What clinical indicators demonstrate improvement in patient comfort?

↓RR, ↓ in muscle activity & sync. w/vent

63. What measures can be taken to ensure patient comfort when the clinical indicators are absent?

refitting mask, coach pt. adjust settings

64. What tidal volume range should be used with NIV?

5-7 ml/kg

65. How is volume manipulated on noninvasive ventilators?

↑ IPAP & EPAP difference

66. Clinical improvement should be noticeable when the patient can tolerate how much time on the NIV?

4-6 hrs.

67. When should attempts at the use of NIV be terminated in favor of more invasive measures?

PH & CO₂ worsen; resp. distress, ↓ O₂

68. What factors affect aerosol delivery during NIV?

SVN or MDI, leak port position, IPAP/EPAP levels, humidifier

69. What problems do nasal masks or full face masks present during aerosol delivery?

air leaks cause continuous flow

70. Complications from NIV are usually due to what three factors?

mask discomfort, air pressure & gas flow

71. What causes eye irritation with NIV and what can be done to alleviate it?

excess air leaks → change/secure mask

72. What causes pressure sores on the nasal bridge and what can be done to alleviate this problem?

straps too tight change mask

73. When using a mouthpiece or lip seal what may be done to reduce leakage of air from the nose?

nose clips

74. What can be done to reduce gastric insufflation?

administration of simethicone agents

75. List the five most serious complications of NIV.
a. aspiration pneumonia
b. mucus plugging
c. hypoxemia
d. hypotension
e. respiratory arrest

76. What are the common methods of weaning a patient from NIV?

reducing IPAP

CRITICAL THINKING QUESTIONS

1. What situation would cause a noninvasive positive pressure ventilator **not** to trigger from expiratory positive airway pressure (EPAP) to inspiratory positive airway pressure breathing (IPAP) or cycle from IPAP to EPAP?

2. What are the issues that lead to patient noncompliance with NIV and how can they be alleviated?

3. Describe how placement of the leak port and oxygen bleed-in affects the F_IO_2 delivered to the patient through NIV.

Chapter **19** **Basic Concepts of Noninvasive Positive Pressure Ventilation**

Case Study 1

A 62-year-old male is currently in the emergency department (ED) being seen for what appears to be an exacerbation of congestive heart failure. He is oriented to person, place, and time but is very anxious. Physical examination findings are as follows: pulse 129 and thready, blood pressure 108/64, temperature 37° C; respirations are 28 breaths/min, shallow, and labored, with accessory muscle use. Auscultation reveals bilateral decreased breath sounds with diffuse coarse crackles on inspiration. The patient has no cough and is diaphoretic. The respiratory therapist places the patient on a nonrebreather mask and draws an arterial blood gas after fifteen minutes. The ABG shows: pH 7.31; $PaCO_2$ 49 mm Hg; PaO_2 53 mm Hg; SaO_2 86%; HCO_3^- 23 mEq/L.

1. Does this patient meet the selection criteria for NIV? Why or why not?

_____

_____

_____

_____

2. If NIV is appropriate, what settings should be used? If not, what other respiratory therapy should be initiated?

_____

_____

_____

After 3 hours of treatment, the patient has become agitated, confused, and uncooperative.

3. What action should be taken at this time?

_____

_____

_____

Case Study 2

A 75-year-old man with a long history of COPD and a past smoking history of 114 pack-years presents to the ED with shortness of breath, productive cough with green purulent sputum, and cyanosis. He has had two prior hospitalizations for acute infective exacerbations of his COPD within the past year. He has no comorbidities or occupational exposure. Physical exam reveals the following: pulse 105 and regular; blood pressure 140/85; respirations 30 with prolonged expiration and use of accessory muscles; percussion is hyperresonant; breath sounds are reduced bilaterally with prolonged expiratory wheezes. Lab work shows WBC 11,500 cells/mm³, room air ABG pH 7.30, $PaCO_2$ 55 mm Hg, PaO_2 53 mm Hg, HCO_3^- 32 mEq/L.

1. Analyze this situation and identify and explain five presenting problems.

_____

_____

_____

_____

_____

2. What treatment recommendations should be suggested for this patient at this time?

_____

_____

_____

_____

_____

A repeat ABG following appropriate therapy reveals the following: pH 7.19, $PaCO_2$ 67 mm Hg, PaO_2 60 mm Hg.

3. What is the most appropriate treatment option at this time?

_____

_____

_____

1. Symptoms of chronic hypoventilation include which of the following?
   1. Fatigue
   2. Morning headache
   3. Hypoxemia
   4. Insomnia
   a. 1 and 2
   b. 2 and 3
   c. 3 and 4
   d. 1 and 4

2. A male COPD patient, 5 ft 10 in tall, has been placed on NIV with an IPAP of 8 cm H_2O and an EPAP of 4 cm H_2O. The patient's exhaled volume was measured at 350 mL and the ABGs on this setting were pH 7.27, $PaCO_2$ 77 mm Hg, PaO_2 50 mm Hg, and base excess +7. The most appropriate action is which of the following?
   a. Increase EPAP to 6 cm H_2O
   b. Increase IPAP to 10 cm H_2O
   c. Decrease IPAP to 6 cm H_2O
   d. Bleed in 4 L/min of oxygen

3. The target tidal volume for a patient with an ideal body weight of 58 kg who is receiving NIV is which of the following?
   a. 250 mL
   b. 350 mL
   c. 500 mL
   d. 700 mL

4. The respiratory therapist notices that there has been a drop in the exhaled tidal volume of a patient receiving NIV. The most appropriate action to take is which of the following?
   a. Increase the IPAP
   b. Decrease the EPAP
   c. Adjust the interface
   d. Change the tubing

5. A patient with chronic hypercapnic respiratory failure is currently using NIV only at night, with the following parameters: assist mode, IPAP 9 cm H_2O and EPAP 4 cm H_2O. The patient is noted to be short of breath with a spontaneous rate of 25 breaths/min. The action that will alleviate this problem is which of the following?
   a. Switch to the control mode.
   b. Increase the IPAP percentage to 35%.
   c. Decrease the EPAP to 2 cm H_2O.
   d. Increase the IPAP to 11 cm H_2O.

6. Which of the following situations will provide the highest oxygen concentration to a patient who is using a portable PTV?
   a. Low IPAP and EPAP settings
   b. High IPAP and EPAP settings
   c. Leak port and oxygen bleed-in at the mask
   d. Leak port and oxygen bleed-in in the circuit

7. The most appropriate type of humidifier to use with NIV is which of the following?
   a. Wick-type humidifier
   b. Heat moisture exchanger
   c. Heated bubble humidifier
   d. Heated passover-type humidifier

8. Which of the following will reduce a significant air leak through the mouth of a patient who is receiving NIV via a nose mask?
   a. Using a chin strap
   b. Adding a forehead spacer
   c. Switching to nasal pillows
   d. Tightening the headgear straps

9. A patient is receiving mask CPAP with 8 cm H_2O and 80% oxygen. The ABG on this setting is pH 7.37, $PaCO_2$ 37 mm Hg, and PaO_2 55 mm Hg. The most appropriate recommendation is which of the following?
   a. Increase the F_IO_2 to 90%.
   b. Intubate and mechanically ventilate.
   c. Increase the CPAP level to 12 cm H_2O.
   d. Switch to bi-level positive pressure ventilation.

10. A patient with which of the following problems should be excluded from a trial with NIV?
    a. Amyotrophic lateral sclerosis
    b. Cardiogenic pulmonary edema
    c. Hemodynamically unstable ARDS
    d. Community-acquired pneumonia

Chapter **19** **Basic Concepts of Noninvasive Positive Pressure Ventilation**

21 Long-Term Ventilation

LEARNING OBJECTIVES

Upon completion of this chapter, the reader will be able to do the following:

1. State the goals of mechanical ventilation in a home environment.
2. List the criteria for selection of patients suitable for successful home care ventilation.
3. Name the factors used to estimate the cost of home mechanical ventilation.
4. Describe facilities used for the care of patients requiring extended ventilator management in terms of type of care provided and cost.
5. Identify the factors used when considering selection of a ventilator for home use.
6. Compare the criteria for discharging a child versus discharging an adult who is ventilator dependent.
7. Explain the use of the following noninvasive ventilation techniques: pneumobelt, chest cuirass, full-body chamber (tank ventilator), and body suit (jacket ventilator).
8. List follow-up assessment techniques used with home-ventilated patients.
9. Describe some of the difficulties families experience when caring for a patient in the home.
10. Identify pieces of equipment that are essential to accomplishing intermittent positive pressure ventilation (IPPV) in the home.
11. Name the specific equipment needed for patients in the home who cannot be without ventilator support.
12. Name the appropriate modes used with first-generation portable/home care ventilators.
13. On the basis of a patient's assessment and ventilator parameters, name the operational features required for that patient's home ventilator and any additional equipment that will be needed.
14. Discuss the instructions given to the patient and caregivers when preparing a patient for discharge home.
15. List the items that should appear in a monthly report of patients on home mechanical ventilation.
16. Describe patients who would benefit from continuous positive airway pressure by nasal mask or pillows.
17. Recommend solutions to potential complications and side effects of nasal mask continuous positive airway pressure.

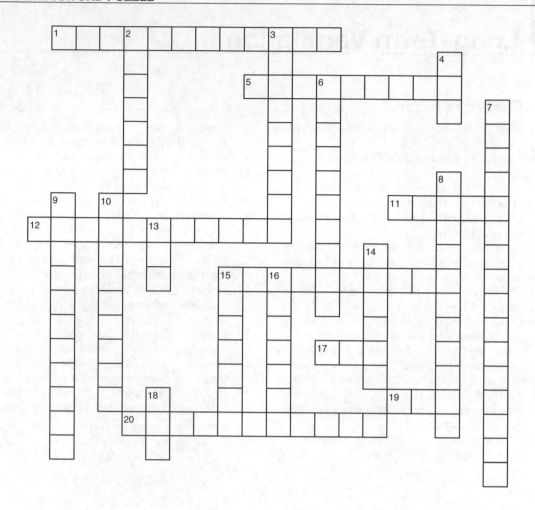

Across

1 Easy to understand and manipulate (two words)
5 Reflux can cause this to erode.
11 Failure of appropriate forward movement of bowel contents
12 Removal of the tracheostomy tube
17 Home care equipment supplier (abbreviation)
19 Mechanical cough machine (abbreviation)
20 Type of tube that goes into the stomach

Down

2 Temporary relief for the caregiver
3 Type of planning team
4 Type of sleep disorder (abbreviation)
6 Intermittent abdominal pressure ventilator
7 Type of breathing used to assist patients with poor respiratory muscle strength
8 Type of TT with an extra opening.
9 Surgical opening between the jejunum and the surface of the abdominal wall
10 Type of speaking valve (two words)
13 Opposite of PPV (abbreviation)
14 Name of a speaking TT
15 Home care disinfectant
16 Type of ventilation indicated in 13 down
18 Ventilator-assisted individuals (abbreviation)

CHAPTER REVIEW QUESTION

1. List the overall goals of long-term home mechanical ventilation.

_____

_____

_____

_____

2. What is considered improvement in psychosocial well-being for a long-term ventilator patient?

_____

3. What are the criteria for a patient to be classified as "chronic ventilator-dependent"?

_____

_____

4. What are the two general categories of patients who require long-term mechanical ventilation?

   a. _____

   b. _____

5. What are the three main criteria that are assessed when evaluating a patient for home mechanical ventilation?

   a. _____

   b. _____

   c. _____

6. What types of patients are most likely to be successful with long-term ventilation?

_____

_____

_____

_____

7. What clinical factors must be considered prior to recommending a patient for long-term mechanical ventilation in the home or in a long-term care facility?

_____

_____

8. What additional criteria must be considered for a child to be considered for home mechanical ventilation?

_____

_____

_____

9. Of the various sites available, a patient who has required mechanical ventilation for over 30 days and who requires intravenous therapy would best be treated in which type of facility?

_____

10. Name the factors that must be considered when estimating a patient's cost of home mechanical ventilation:

_____

_____

_____

_____

11. In order of cost (most expensive to least expensive), list the potential locations for patients who require long-term ventilatory care:

_____

_____

12. List the five most important factors when choosing a ventilator for home use:

   a. _____

   b. _____

   c. _____

   d. _____

   e. _____

13. What backup equipment is necessary for a patient requiring long-term mechanical ventilation at home? What is the rationale for each?

Backup Equipment	Rationale
_____	_____
_____	_____
_____	_____

14. What is the rationale for the increased level of follow-up and evaluation of the ventilatory status of children maintained on mechanical ventilation at home as compared to adults?

_____

_____

15. Identify the three classifications of ventilator-dependent patients

   a. _____

   b. _____

   c. _____

16. Identify the psychosocial factors that must be addressed to ensure a successful transition home for the ventilator-dependent patient.

_____

_____

_____

_____

17. What factors must be addressed when evaluating the home environment prior to discharge of patients requiring mechanical ventilation?

_____

_____

_____

18. Discuss what difficulties family members experience when caring for a patient in the home.

_____

_____

_____

19. In addition to the mechanical ventilator and its related equipment, list some of the other equipment/supplies that are needed to support the patient receiving mechanical ventilation in the home.

_____

_____

_____

_____

_____

_____

20. List the three electrical power sources used by home ventilators.

a. _____

b. _____

c. _____

21. Compare the three types of negative-pressure ventilators:

Ventilator	Advantages	Disadvantages
Iron Lung		
Chest Cuirass		
Body Suit		

22. List the contraindications for the use of negative-pressure ventilators:

_____

_____

_____

23. What is the main disadvantage of placing a patient in the intermittent mandatory ventilation (IMV) mode when using an earlier model (first-generation) home care ventilator?

_____

24. Explain why a patient receiving mechanical ventilation with oxygen and positive end-expiratory pressure (PEEP) in the home may encounter difficulty triggering the ventilator?

_____

_____

_____

25. What are some of the advantages of providing home mechanical ventilation with the newer (second-generation) portable home care ventilators?

_____

_____

_____

_____

26. What three complications are common to both long-term and critically ill patients who require mechanical ventilation?

a. _____

b. _____

c. _____

27. Compare the modes available on the first-generation portable/home care ventilators with the second-generation ventilators.

First Generation	Second Generation
_____	_____
_____	_____
_____	_____

28. List the four most common gastrointestinal disorders associated with patients receiving long-term mechanical ventilation.

a. _____

b. _____

c. _____

d. _____

29. A substantial number of patients who transfer to long-term care facilities on mechanical ventilation have what type of disorders?

_____

30. List the factors that contribute to psychological problems in ventilator-assisted individuals.

_____

_____

31. How do the rocking bed and pneumobelt support spontaneous ventilation?

_____

_____

32. The rocking bed should not be used for patients with what conditions?

_____

_____

33. What type of patient would benefit from a rocking bed as a form of ventilatory support?

_____

34. In what type of therapy is the phrenic nerve stimulated through surgically implanted electrodes?

_____

35. What is the most common form of respiratory therapy used to treat obstructive sleep apnea (OSA)?

_____

36. What happens to an OSA patient during sleep?

_____

37. List the goals of continuous positive airway pressure (CPAP) therapy when used to treat OSA.

_____

_____

_____

38. What patient interfaces are available for delivering CPAP therapy?

_____

_____

39. List two major advantages associated with newer home CPAP units.

   a. _____

   b. _____

40. What are the complications associated with CPAP therapy?

   _____

   _____

   _____

41. What are the physical requirements a patient needs to perform glossopharyngeal breathing?

   _____

   _____

42. What type of patients benefit from the use of glossopharyngeal breathing?

   _____

43. What are the minimum vital capacity (VC) and peak cough expiratory flow rate (PCEF) necessary to produce an effective cough?

   _____

44. List three techniques that aid in management of secretions for patients with neuromuscular disease:

   a. _____

   b. _____

   c. _____

45. How is assisted coughing performed?

   _____

   _____

46. What are the advantages of mechanical insufflation-exsufflation (MI-E) as compared to tracheal suctioning?

   _____

   _____

47. In what type of patients is MI-E contraindicated?

   _____

   _____

48. What type of tracheostomy tube should a therapist recommend for a patient who is unable to speak and at risk of aspiration?

   _____

49. What type of tracheostomy tube should a therapist recommend for a patient who has no trouble swallowing and can breathe for long periods of time?

   _____

50. Why is it important that children with tracheostomies have their language and vocal skills evaluated?

   _____

   _____

51. In addition to deflating the cuff, what ventilator parameters can be adjusted to help a patient produce speech to or improve speech quality?

   _____

   _____

52. What are the potential hazards of cuff deflation of VAIs?

   _____

53. Before a cuff is deflated to allow for speaking, what should the patient be evaluated for?

   _____

54. What devices are available to allow VAIs to speak?

   _____

   _____

55. How does a Passy-Muir speaking valve allow for speech in the patient with a tracheostomy who is receiving mechanical ventilation?

   _____

   _____

56. List the circumstances in which the use of speaking devices may be contraindicated:

   _____

   _____

   _____

   _____

   _____

57. Compare the functions of the Portex and the Pittsburg speaking tracheostomy tubes.

_____

_____

_____

_____

58. What steps need to be taken prior to setting up a speaking valve for a VAI?

_____

_____

_____

_____

59. What is the most cost-effective disinfecting solution available for home care patients to disinfect their equipment?

_____

60. How long must water be boiled before it can be used in a humidifier?

_____

61. Prior to discharge, what are the primary skills the respiratory therapist must teach the patient, his or her family, and others involved in the care of the patient?

_____

_____

_____

62. What components must be included in a written monthly report when performing a home visit?

_____

_____

_____

CRITICAL THINKING QUESTIONS

Questions 1 and 2 refer to the following scenario:

After undergoing a sleep study, a patient diagnosed with obstructive sleep apnea (OSA) is prescribed CPAP via nasal mask. During a follow-up visit by the therapist, the patient states that his sleep is not improving and that he is experiencing eye irritation.

1. What could be the cause of the patient's problem?

_____

_____

2. What steps can the therapist take to alleviate the situation?

_____

_____

Question 3 refers to the following scenario:

A ventilator-dependent patient in a long-term care facility is being maintained on pressure support ventilation. The respiratory therapist is asked to evaluate the patient to see if he can tolerate a speaking valve. After cuff deflation, and prior to attaching the valve, the patient suddenly becomes short of breath, with an increase in heart rate.

3. What could have brought on the sudden onset of respiratory distress?

_____

_____

_____

_____

Question 4 refers to the following scenario:

Fifteen minutes after initiating PEEP with an external threshold resistor for a patient supported by a home care ventilator, the respiratory therapist observes that the patient's respiratory rate has doubled, her tidal volume has dropped significantly, and the ventilator's low pressure alarm has been activated.

4. What is the probable cause of this problem?

_____

CASE STUDIES

Case Study 1

A patient in the early stages of a neuromuscular disease complains to his physician that he is having difficulty sleeping. In addition, he is experiencing headaches and becomes increasingly tired towards the end of the day.

1. What are the possible causes of this patient's symptoms?

_____

2. What type of therapy should the therapist recommend to help treat this patient?

_____

3. What would be the goals of the recommended therapy?

_____

4. How would you evaluate the effectiveness of the therapy?

_____

Case Study 2

A 70-year-old female had spent 1 month in the hospital for exacerbation of COPD. After numerous attempts at weaning had failed, the patient received a tracheostomy. After careful evaluation, the patient was discharged home on continuous ventilatory support. A follow-up visit was made 2 weeks post discharge. The therapist found the patient to be febrile, auscultation revealed rhonchi in the right upper and middle lobes, and suctioning produced a moderate amount of yellow sputum. The patient was admitted to the hospital and diagnosed with pneumonia.

1. What would be your assessment of why this patient developed a pulmonary infection so soon after discharge?

   _____

   _____

2. What recommendations, if any, would you make?

   _____

   _____

NBRC-STYLE QUESTIONS

1. If a home care ventilator does not have an F_IO_2 control, what is the most common means by which oxygen can be delivered to the patient?
   a. An external blender
   b. Using a microprocessor-controlled proportioning valve
   c. Mixing air and oxygen cylinders to approximate the desired F_IO_2
   d. Bleeding oxygen into the system through the inspiratory limb

2. In the home setting, how long should suction catheters be soaked in a disinfectant solution?
   a. A minimum of 2 minutes
   b. A minimum of 5 minutes
   c. A minimum of 10 minutes
   d. A minimum of 25 minutes

3. Which of the following represents the range of CPAP levels available on most home care units?
   a. 0 to 2.0 cm H_2O
   b. 2.5 to 20 cm H_2O
   c. 25 to 35 cm H_2O
   d. 35 to 45 cm H_2O

4. All of the following patient conditions can be treated with negative-pressure ventilation *except*:
   a. Excessive secretions
   b. Neuromuscular disease
   c. Spinal cord injuries
   d. Central hypoventilation syndromes

5. During a follow-up visit of a patient recently started on CPAP therapy by nasal mask, the patient complains of nasal dryness and congestion. Which of the following recommendations would help remedy the problem?
   a. Decrease the flow rate
   b. Decrease the level of CPAP
   c. Add humidification or recommend use of a nasal spray
   d. Readjust the mask to correct for any leaks

6. All of the following are generally part of a monthly home evaluation except?
   a. Vital signs
   b. Pulse oximetry
   c. Bedside pulmonary function studies
   d. Arterial blood gas

7. Contraindications to long-term home mechanical ventilation include:
   a. An F_IO_2 requirement > 30%
   b. PEEP > 5 cm H_2O
   c. The need for continuous invasive monitoring
   d. The need for frequent secretion removal

8. Which of the following conditions allow(s) patients certain periods of spontaneous breathing during the day, and generally require(s) only nocturnal ventilatory support?
   1. Myasthenia gravis
   2. End-stage COPD
   3. Kyphoscoliosis
   4. Multiple sclerosis
   a. 1 only
   b. 3 and 4
   c. 1, 3, and 4
   d. 1, 2, 3, and 4

9. Patient assessment prior to decannulation should include which of the following?
   1. Airway patency
   2. Sufficient muscle strength to generate a cough
   3. Volume and thickness of secretions
   4. Sleep studies
   a. 1 only
   b. 1 and 4
   c. 1, 2, and 3
   d. 1, 2, 3, and 4

10. All of the following are realistic goals of home mechanical ventilation except:
    a. To reverse the disease process
    b. To improve quality of life
    c. To prolong life
    d. To reduce the number of hospitalizations

22 Neonatal and Pediatric Mechanical Ventilation

LEARNING OBJECTIVES

Upon completion of this chapter, the reader will be able to do the following:

1. Discuss the clinical manifestations of respiratory distress in neonatal and pediatric patients.
2. Identify differences in the level of noninvasive ventilatory support.
3. Describe device function and settings for different mechanical respiratory support strategies.
4. Identify the primary and secondary goals of ventilatory support of newborn and pediatric patients.
5. Explain some key areas of assessment that influence the decision on whether to initiate ventilatory support.
6. Recognize the indications, goals, limitations, and potentially harmful effects of continuous positive airway pressure (CPAP) in a clinical case.
7. Describe the basic design of nasal devices used to deliver CPAP to an infant.
8. Compare and contrast a mechanical ventilator equipped with a CPAP delivery system to a freestanding CPAP system.
9. From patient data, recognize the need for mechanical ventilatory support in newborn and pediatric patients.
10. Identify the essential features of a neonatal and pediatric mechanical ventilator.
11. Explain how the advanced features of a ventilator enhance its usefulness over a wide range of clinical settings.
12. Relate the major differences between older-generation neonatal ventilators and modern microprocessor-controlled mechanical ventilators.
13. Distinguish demand flow from continuous flow, and discuss other modifications that have been made to the basic infant ventilator.
14. Select appropriate ventilator settings based on the patient's weight, diagnosis, and clinical history; also discuss strategies and rationale for ventilator settings.
15. Discuss newborn and pediatric applications, technical aspects, patient management, and cautions for the following ventilatory modes: pressure-control ventilation, volume-control ventilation, dual-controlled ventilation, pressure support ventilation, airway pressure release ventilation, and neurally adjusted ventilatory assist.
16. Discuss the rationale and indications for high-frequency ventilation in newborn and pediatric patients.
17. Compare the characteristics and basic delivery systems of the following high-frequency ventilation techniques: high-frequency positive pressure ventilation, high-frequency jet ventilation, high-frequency flow interruption, high-frequency percussive ventilation, and high-frequency oscillatory ventilation.
18. Explain the physiologic and theoretic mechanisms of gas exchange that govern high-frequency ventilation, and defend the mechanism believed to be most correct.
19. Explain how settings of a given high-frequency technique are initially adjusted, the effect of individual controls on gas exchange, and strategies of patient management.
20. Discuss the physiologic benefits of inhaled nitric oxide (NO) therapy, and suggest recommended treatment strategies.

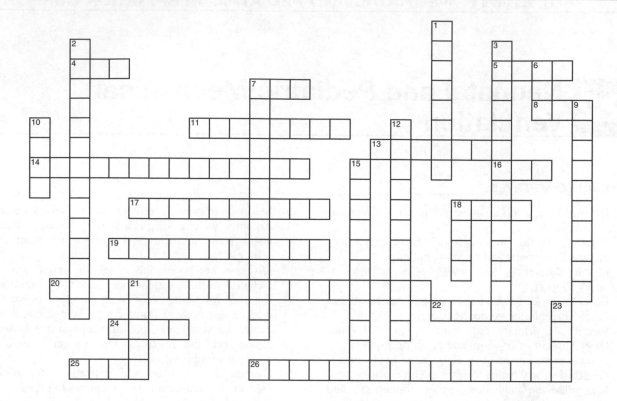

Across

4 Condition that is responsive to 24 across (abbreviation)

5 Type of ventilation that uses the highest rates (8 to 20 Hz) (abbreviation)

7 Pulmonary disease of infants; high airway resistance is a major component (abbreviation)

8 Neonatal problem commonly treated with methylxanthines (abbreviation)

11 Type of aspiration syndrome that occurs in term or postterm neonates

13 Abnormal tubelike passage between the trachea and the esophagus

14 A deficiency in the cartilage around a bronchus; leads to atelectasis

16 Infant who weighs 1500 to 2500 g (abbreviation)

17 Type of heart disease that is present at birth

18 Mode that is unique to infant mechanical ventilation (abbreviation)

19 Congenital split of the roof of the mouth (two words)

20 Incomplete embryological formation of the diaphragm leads to this. (two words)

22 Type of hemoglobin present in a fetus

24 Noninvasive method of increasing functional residual capacity (FRC) and improving lung compliance

25 Mode of ventilation used to percuss the chest to remove secretions (abbreviation)

26 Structure that may remain open after birth (two words)

Down

1 Brand of surfactant replacement

2 Softening of the cartilages of the trachea

3 Failure of the nasopharyngeal septum to rupture causes this malformation. (two words)

6 This is usually treated by 24 across. (abbreviation)

7 Viral infection that causes inflammation, swelling, and airway obstruction

9 Exchange of gas between lung units with different time constants

10 Infant weighing less than 1500 g (abbreviation)

12 Used to improve pulmonary blood flow and enhance arterial oxygenation (two words)

15 Interface most often used for application of 24 across (two words)

18 Historically, the mode most often used for infants (abbreviation)

21 Mode that uses frequencies up to 150 breaths/min (abbreviation)

23 An invasive life support procedure (abbreviation)

1. Name the three basic types of devices involved in the mechanical ventilation of newborn and pediatric patients.

    a. _____

    b. _____

    c. _____

2. What concepts must a clinician taking care of the neonatal and pediatric population understand?

    _____

    _____

    _____

3. Define the term *respiratory failure*.

    _____

4. Respiratory failure in a neonate is characterized by what laboratory and clinical data?

    _____

    _____

    _____

    _____

5. List the five factors that make neonatal and pediatric patients more vulnerable to rapid deterioration.

    a. _____

    b. _____

    c. _____

    d. _____

    e. _____

6. List the signs or respiratory distress in the neonate.

    _____

    _____

    _____

    _____

    _____

7. What can cause premature neonates to become apneic?

    _____

8. How can tissue oxygenation be assessed physically?

    _____

    _____

    _____

9. In what way can oxygen delivery and tissue perfusion be evaluated clinically?

    _____

10. Give two examples of times when a very individualized approach for managing gas exchange during ventilatory support is needed early in the patient's management.

    a. _____

    b. _____

11. List the five goals of mechanical ventilatory support in newborn and pediatric patients.

    a. _____

    b. _____

    c. _____

    d. _____

    e. _____

12. What are the goals of maintaining an appropriate FRC in a newborn or pediatric patient?

    _____

    _____

13. What laboratory data define respiratory failure in newborns?

    _____

14. The minimum acceptable pH for a premature or term newborn is _____.

15. What laboratory data define respiratory failure in pediatric patients?

    _____

16. When maximum oxygen delivery to the tissues is critical, why is fetal hemoglobin not desirable?

    _____

    _____

    _____

17. What are the most common uses for CPAP in pediatric patients?

_____

_____

_____

18. Newborns with what conditions would be good candidates for CPAP?

_____

_____

_____

_____

19. List at least eight indications for CPAP in the neonate.

a. _____

b. _____

c. _____

d. _____

e. _____

f. _____

g. _____

h. _____

20. What six factors constitute the physical examination indicators for the use of CPAP?

a. _____

b. _____

c. _____

d. _____

e. _____

f. _____

21. What are the blood gas values that indicate a need for CPAP?

_____

_____

22. Chest radiographic indications for the use of CPAP include what two findings?

_____

_____

23. List the seven conditions that are thought to respond to CPAP and which are associated with one or more of the previously listed clinical presentations.

a. _____

b. _____

c. _____

d. _____

e. _____

f. _____

g. _____

24. What are the two general approaches used to minimize the use of mechanical ventilation and protect the neonatal respiratory system?

a. _____

b. _____

25. What does InSURE stand for?

_____

26. List at least two incidences where CPAP therapy can be dangerous to an infant.

a. _____

b. _____

27. When may infants require intubation and mechanical ventilation rather than CPAP?

_____

_____

_____

_____

28. Name the three methods of delivering CPAP to newborns.

a. _____

b. _____

c. _____

29. The most commonly used interface for the application of CPAP is _____

30. What are the most critical facts concerning the application of CPAP interfaces?

_____

_____

31. How is the CPAP apparatus stabilized?

_____

_____

32. CPAP stabilizing equipment should be checked periodically for what?

_____

_____

_____

33. List the five components that make up a CPAP system.

a. _____

b. _____

c. _____

d. _____

e. _____

34. List four problems that improper positioning of the nasopharyngeal (NP) tube can cause.

a. _____

b. _____

c. _____

d. _____

35. How is pressure regulated in bubble CPAP machines?

_____

_____

36. What is the initial pressure setting for CPAP and how should the CPAP level be adjusted?

_____

_____

37. What is considered an adequate level of CPAP?

_____

_____

38. List ten possible complications of CPAP.

a. _____

b. _____

c. _____

d. _____

e. _____

f. _____

g. _____

h. _____

i. _____

j. _____

39. Some research suggests that this intervention contributes to the development of bronchopulmonary displagia (BPD) in neonates:

_____

40. List some complications that accompany neonatal endotracheal intubation.

_____

_____

_____

_____

_____

_____

_____

41. List some uses of noninvasive positive pressure ventilation (NIV).

_____

_____

_____

_____

42. How is NIV most commonly applied to neonates?

_____

_____

_____

_____

43. List some suggested initial intermittent mandatory ventilation settings for neonates.

_____

_____

_____

_____

44. Describe SiPAP.

_____

_____

45. What are common SiPAP settings?

_____

_____

_____

46. Complete the following table.

CPAP Application Disorder	CPAP Application Device
4-year-old with juvenile spinal muscle atrophy (Kugelberg-Welander disease)	_____
1-year-old with progressive spinal muscular atrophy of infants (Werdnig-Hoffman paralysis)	_____
10-year-old with obstructive sleep apnea (OSA)	_____
3-year-old with bronchomalacia	_____

47. What are the benefits of BiPAP and NIV in the pediatric population?

_____

_____

48. What are some initial settings for a pediatric patient receiving BiPAP?

_____

_____

_____

49. List the major categories of indications for mechanical ventilation in the neonate.

_____

_____

_____

_____

_____

_____

_____

50. What neurological problems can compromise the central drive of a newborn?

_____

_____

51. List seven diseases/syndromes that can reduce lung compliance and/or increase airway resistance in a neonate.

a. _____

b. _____

c. _____

d. _____

e. _____

f. _____

g. _____

52. List four diseases/syndromes that impair the cardiovascular function of a neonate.

a. _____

b. _____

c. _____

d. _____

53. List the major categories of indications for mechanical ventilation of pediatric patients.

_____

_____

_____

_____

_____

_____

_____

_____

54. What are the indicators of respiratory failure in pediatric patients?

_____

_____

55. List four neuromuscular/hypotonic disorders that are indicators for mechanical ventilation of pediatric patients.

a. _____

b. _____

c. _____

d. _____

56. In the past, the modality that was used more than any other to ventilate infants was: _____.

57. List the essential features of an infant/pediatric ventilator.

_____

_____

_____

_____

_____

_____

_____

_____

_____

58. How do nonessential features enhance a ventilator's usefulness over a wide range of clinical settings?

_____

_____

59. In an infant ventilator, what type of trigger avoids breath stacking and asynchrony?

_____

60. Discuss the difference between continuous flow and demand flow for spontaneous breaths.

_____

_____

61. What triggering methods are available for neonatal and pediatric patients?

_____

_____

62. What is the preferred triggering method for neonates? Why?

_____

_____

63. What is an important advancement made in neonatal and pediatric ventilators?

_____

64. What is the major limitation of proximal flow sensors?

_____

65. Currently, what is the most widely used mode of ventilation in neonates and pediatrics?

_____

66. Describe how peak inspiratory pressure (PIP) can be optimized during manual ventilation.

_____

_____

67. What is the purpose of positive end-expiratory pressure (PEEP)?

_____

68. What are acceptable initial PEEP settings?

_____

69. When should PEEP be increased?

_____

70. What is meant by the term *flow chop?*

_____

71. (a) Calculate the time constant when Raw = 45 cm/H_2O/L/sec and C_L = 0.004 L/cm H_2O.

_____

_____

  (b) What T_I should be set for this time constant?

_____

72. (a) Calculate the time constant when Raw = 30 cm/H_2O/L/sec and C_L = 0.002 L/cm H_2O.

_____

_____

  (b) What T_I should be set for this time constant?

_____

73. What can be done to reduce the potential for ventilator-induced hyperinflation in patients with bronchopulmonary dysplasia or meconium aspiration?

_____

_____

74. What is considered an acceptable leak around a cuffless endotracheal tube (ET)?

_____

75. Calculate the percent leak when V_{Tinsp} = 67 mL and V_{Texh} = 55 mL.

_____

213

76. Mean airway pressures greater than _____ have been associated with lung injury in neonates.

77. What PaO_2 levels should be maintained in neonates and pediatric patients?

_____

_____

78. What parameter is set to ensure a tidal volume during volume-targeted ventilation?

_____

79. What factors determine T_I when VV is used?

_____

_____

80. What types of pediatric patients respond well to volume controlled–intermittent mandatory ventilation (VC-IMV)?

_____

81. The recommended V_T values for pressure-support ventilation (PSV) are: _____

82. What is a cycling problem that can occur during PSV in patients with an ET or tracheostomy tube?

_____

83. The most widely used form of dual-control ventilation in neonates and pediatric patients is:_____

_____

84. Explain how pressure regulated volume control (PRVC) works.

_____

85. Describe how machine volume with volume backing works.

_____

86. Explain how volume-assured pressure support (VAPS) works.

_____

87. What advantage does volume support ventilation (VSV) have over PSV in the administration of surfactant replacement therapy to an infant?

_____

_____

_____

88. How is weaning accomplished in infants with the A/C option?

_____

_____

89. How are the pressure levels set in airway pressure release ventilation (APRV) for neonatal and pediatric patients?

_____

_____

90. What benefits does spontaneous breathing at the highter pressure level during APRV provide?

_____

_____

91. What parameters does NAVA allow the patient to control?

_____

_____

92. What are the goals of lung-protective therapy in the neonatal and pediatric patient?

_____

_____

_____

93. What types of lung-protective strategies may be used during ventilation of neonatal and pediatric patients?

_____

_____

_____

_____

94. When should high-frequency ventilation (HFV) be considered in an infant's clinical course?

_____

_____

_____

_____

95. List three complications from HFV.

a. _____

b. _____

c. _____

96. Complete the following table.

HFV Type	Definition (including frequencies)	Uses

97. Explain the physiological mechanism of gas exchange in HFV.

_____

_____

98. List the preparations that should be completed before a patient is placed on HFV.

_____

_____

_____

_____

Chapter **22** **Neonatal and Pediatric Mechanical Ventilation**

99. What is the general goal for all types of HFV?

_____

_____

100. What do preparations of exogenous surfactant typically contain?

_____

_____

101. Describe the dosing procedure for exogenous surfactant.

_____

_____

_____

_____

_____

102. Name the two types of toxicity that have been reported with application of inhaled NO.

a. _____

b. _____

CRITICAL THINKING QUESTIONS

1. A pediatric patient with a 4-mm ET is receiving PSV. The respiratory therapist notes that inspiration seems to exceed 1 second. What is the most likely cause of this problem and how can it be corrected?

_____

_____

2. VSV has what advantage over PSV during surfactant replacement therapy?

_____

_____

3. An infant receiving nasal CPAP is crying, and each time the infant's mouth opens, the CPAP level on the pressure manometer drops significantly. Why is the pressure dropping and what can be done to correct it?

_____

_____

_____

_____

4. What circumstance can reduce the level of support provided in PRVC? What problems can this lead to?

_____

CASE STUDIES

Case Study 1

A 29 weeks' gestation, 2-hour-old infant is in the neonatal ICU in an oxyhood with an F_IO_2 of 0.5. Physical examination reveals intercostal and substernal retractions, a respiratory rate of 68 breaths/min, and a pulse of 145. The ABG values are as follows: pH = 7.21, $PaCO_2$ = 70 mm Hg, PaO_2 = 41 mm Hg. Manual ventilation of this patient demonstrates bilateral chest movement and aeration at 25 cm H_2O.

1. The most appropriate PIP setting for this patient is:

_____

During mechanical ventilation, the patient's pressure-volume loop changes from that shown in Figure 22-1A to that shown in Figure 22-1B.

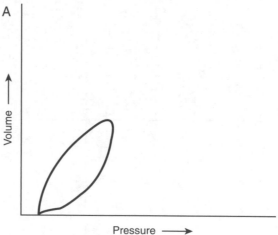

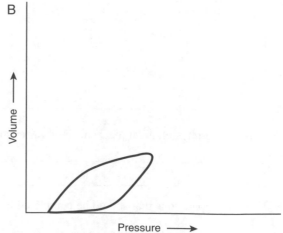

2. What is the most likely cause of this change?

_____

The patient receives Survanta at 2 mL/kg. During this time the ventilator F_IO_2 is increased to 1. Each partial dose is followed by a 30-second period on the ventilator. The pressure-volume loop then takes on the shape shown in Figure 22-2.

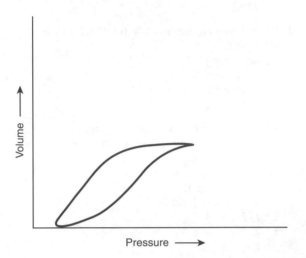

1. What is the most likely cause of this change?

_____

Case Study 2

A newborn male infant weighing 1275 g and approximately 28 weeks' gestation is intubated and receiving mechanical ventilation with TCPL at these settings: rate = 40 breaths/min, PIP = 24 cm H_2O, PEEP = 4 cm H_2O, F_IO_2 = 0.75. The patient received Survanta about 1 hour ago. The ABG results after surfactant therapy were these: pH = 7.36, $PaCO_2$ = 38 mm Hg, PaO_2 = 80 mm Hg. The infant is pink and active; the pulse oximeter reads 96%.

1. What would be the most appropriate action in this situation?

_____

Over the next 2 hours, the patient's oxygen saturations begin to decline and his oxygen requirements increase. Breath sounds are bilaterally diminished, the pulse oximeter reading is 86% with an F_IO_2 of 0.55, and the patient is agitated. The respiratory therapist suctions the patient, but no improvement is noted.

2. Name the two most likely causes of this patient's distress.

_____

_____

3. What is the most appropriate action at this time?

_____

_____

Case Study 3

A 24 weeks' gestation neonate weighing 730 g had no signs of respirations and had central cyanosis at birth. He was intubated in the delivery room and transported to the neonatal ICU. He had poor gas exchange during manual resuscitation, and the decision was made to place him on HFOV.

1. What should be the setting for the mean airway pressure?

_____

2. The initial frequency setting should be _____ Hz.

3. How should the initial pressure gradient be set?

_____

NBRC–STYLE QUESTIONS

1. Which of the following is the best method of ensuring an effective CPAP system?
   a. Use of audible and visual alarm systems
   b. Incorporation of F_IO_2 and pressure monitors
   c. Careful monitoring of the patient's WOB and oxygenation status
   d. Use only of a mechanical ventilator with continuous flow capability

2. The type of CPAP delivery system that produces vibrations that may have a beneficial effect is which of the following?
   a. Bubble CPAP
   b. Freestanding CPAP device
   c. Mechanical ventilators with CPAP settings
   d. Improvised freestanding CPAP delivery device

3. The safest and most effective method of CPAP delivery to a newborn is with which of the following?
   a. Vapotherm
   b. Hamilton Arabella
   c. Fisher & Paykel bubble CPAP
   d. Improvised freestanding CPAP device

4. In newborns, PEEP is used to accomplish which of the following?
   1. Recruit alveoli
   2. Prevent atelectasis
   3. Decrease compliance
   4. Establish functional residual capacity
   a. 1 and 3
   b. 1 and 2
   c. 3 and 4
   d. 2 and 4

Chapter **22** **Neonatal and Pediatric Mechanical Ventilation**

5. The disease state that prolongs time constants is which of the following?
   a. Acute lung injury
   b. Apnea of prematurity
   c. Bronchopulmonary dysplasia
   d. Respiratory distress syndrome

6. A newborn is currently in an oxygen hood with an F_IO_2 of 0.7. The patient's ABG values are these: pH = 7.31, $PaCO_2$ = 49 mm Hg, PaO_2 = 50 mm Hg. The most appropriate action is to initiate which of the following?
   a. PSV
   b. CPAP
   c. TPV
   d. SIMV

7. A neonate receiving nasal CPAP of 8 cm H_2O with an F_IO_2 of 0.65 has the following ABG values: pH = 7.2, $PaCO_2$ = 69 mm Hg, and PaO_2 = 48 mm Hg. The most appropriate action is which of the following?
   a. Increase the F_IO_2 to 0.75
   b. Increase CPAP to 10 cm H_2O
   c. Change to nasopharyngeal CPAP
   d. Intubate and mechanically ventilate with pressure controlled-intermittent mandatory ventilation (PC-IMV)

8. Before an infant is put on PC-IMV, the PIP should be determined by which of the following methods?
   a. Estimate the PIP for the patient, set the value at a level higher than this, and adjust downward
   b. Compare chest movement and bilateral aeration to the PIP during manual ventilation
   c. Estimate the PIP for the patient, set the value at a level lower than this, and adjust upward as needed
   d. Set the PIP to a safe level, attach the patient to the ventilator, and monitor for improvement in overall appearance and oxygen saturation

9. Calculate the patient's estimated V_T in PC-IMV when T_I is 0.5 second and flow is 8.75 L/min.
   a. 54 mL
   b. 62 mL
   c. 73 mL
   d. 95 mL

10. V_T is increased during PCV by which of the following?
    a. Increasing PIP
    b. Increasing PEEP
    c. Decreasing flow rate
    d. Increasing T_I

11. Which of the following must be monitored during administration of surfactant replacements?
    1. Heart rate
    2. Oxygenation
    3. Temperature
    4. Airway patency
    a. 1, 2, and 4
    b. 2, 3, and 4
    c. 1 and 3
    d. 1, 2, 3, and 4

23 Special Techniques in Ventilatory Support

LEARNING OBJECTIVES

Upon completion of this chapter, the reader will be able to do the following:

1. Discuss the benefits and disadvantages of airway pressure-release ventilation (APRV)
2. Recommend initial settings for initiating APRV in patients with acute lung injury (ALI)/acute respiratory distress syndrome (ARDS).
3. Explain how the controls operate with the SensorMedics 3100B oscillator.
4. Recommend initial ventilator settings for an adult with the 3100B unit.
5. List types of medications that may be used in transitioning from volume-control continuous mandatory ventilation (VC-CMV) to high-frequency oscillatory ventilation (HFOV) settings.
6. Explain how the chest wiggle factor is influenced by HFOV settings.
7. Name pulmonary pathological conditions in which heliox therapy may be beneficial.
8. Compare the differences between set tidal volume (V_T), monitored V_{TT}, and actual V_T delivery during heliox therapy.
9. Describe how heliox used with a mechanical ventilator may affect pressures and fractional inspired oxygen concentration (F_IO_2) monitoring and delivery.
10. Explain how to set up heliox cylinders with a mechanical ventilator.
11. Name at least four techniques that can help determine the correct placement of the esophageal EDI catheter.
12. Provide examples of how the EDI waveform can be of value in monitoring critically ill patients.
13. Discuss various factors that can cause a low EDI signal and a high EDI signal.
14. Describe the safety backup features and alarms available with neutrally adjusted ventilator assist (NAVA).
15. Calculate an estimated pressure delivery when given the NAVA level, EDI peak, EDI minimum, and positive end-expiratory pressure (PEEP).
16. Explain what parameters (pressure, flow, volume, neural signal, time) are used to deliver a breath during NAVA ventilation.
17. Identify clinical situations in which NAVA should be used.

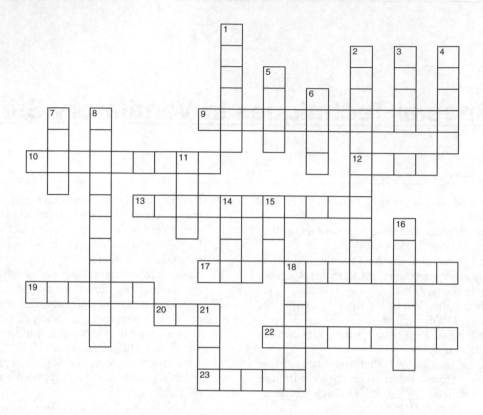

Across

9 Region of the lung that receives the most ventilation
10 HFOV control that influences $PaCO_2$
12 Mode of ventilation with two levels of continuous positive airway pressure (CPAP) (abbreviation)
13 Factor observed from the level of the clavicle to the midthigh during HFOV (two words)
17 HFOV's equivalent to PEEP (abbreviation)
18 First parameter set in starting HFOV (two words)
19 Helium-oxygen mixture
20 Technique that allows the gas flow to each lung to be controlled separately (abbreviation)
22 Region of the lung receiving the best blood flow
23 A property of helium

Down

1 Forward and backward excursion of this helps determine V_T
2 Type of breathing allowed during biphasic CPAP
3 Type of flow waveform produced by HFOV
4 Cycles per minute
5 HFOV is used in the management of this pulmonary problem. (abbreviation)
6 HFOV control that directly affects PaO_2 (abbreviation)
7 Heart-lung bypass machine (abbreviation)
8 Brief interval at P_{low} (two words)
11 Type of ET used to accomplish 20 across (abbreviation)
14 Repair of this may cause unilateral lung injury (abbreviation)
15 Applies internal percussion to the lungs (abbreviation)
16 Biphasic CPAP on the Covidien Nellcor Puritan Bennett 840 (two words)
18 Biphasic CPAP on the SERVO^i (two words)
21 This can be avoided by starting HFOV early in patients with severe acute lung injury/acute respiratory distress syndrome (ALI/ARDS). (abbreviation)

CHAPTER REVIEW QUESTIONS

1. Define *APRV*.

_____

_____

_____

_____

2. Refer to the APRV waveform in the following figure.

Time (seconds)

(a) What is the P_{low}? _____

(b) What is the P_{high}? _____

(c) What is the T_{low}? _____

(d) What is the T_{high}? _____

3. In APRV, the trigger and cycle variables when the patient does not breathe are:_____

_____

4. Give two other names for APRV that are used in the United States.

a. _____

b. _____

5. List the physiological and hemodynamic advantages of APRV compared with other forms of ventilation.

_____

_____

_____

_____

_____

6. List the main disadvantages of APRV.

_____

_____

_____

_____

7. Calculate the APRV respiratory rate that would deliver a P_{low} for 0.75 second and a P_{high} for 4.75 seconds.

_____

_____

_____

8. In APRV, $\dot{V}_E$ depends on what two factors?

_____

_____

9. The range for the P_{high} setting is _____.

10. Why would a practitioner want to set the P_{low} setting at $0\,cm\,H_2O$?

_____

11. The range for the T_{high} setting is _____.

12. How should the T_{low} setting be chosen?

_____

_____

_____

13. For a patient with ARDS, the typical range for the T_{low} setting is _____.

14. Ventilation and $PaCO_2$ are determined by what three factors?

a. _____

b. _____

c. _____

15. Describe one method of weaning a patient from APRV.

_____

_____

_____

_____

16. HFOV oscillates the lungs at what rates?

_____

17. What creates the high-frequency oscillations in the SensorMedics 3100B?

_____

18. What type of flow waveform is created during HFOV?

_____

19. What determines V_T during HFOV?

_____

_____

20. What determines the appropriateness of the power setting?

_____

_____

21. Increasing the HFOV frequency does what to patient ventilation? Why?

_____

22. Reducing the HFOV frequency does what to patient ventilation? Why?

_____

23. What does the $T_I\%$ represent on the SensorMedics 3100B?

_____

_____

24. How does the bias flow setting influence the patient's $PaCO_2$?

_____

_____

_____

25. Complete the following HFOV table.

Control	Brief Description	Typical/Initial Setting
mP_{aw}		
Amplitude		
Frequency		
$T_I\%$		
Bias flow		
F_IO_2		

26. Describe the function of each of the valves on the SensorMedics 3100B.

_____

_____

_____

27. List the indications for HFOV in adults.

_____

_____

_____

28. What is the one exclusion criterion for use of the SensorMedics 3100B?

_____

29. List the types of medications that may be used in transitioning from VC-CMV to HFOV in an adult.

_____

_____

30. A patient on HFOV may be checked for a return to conventional ventilation when what two parameters have been reached?

_____

31. What two ventilator modes are favored for returning a patient to conventional ventilation after HFOV?

_____

32. Describe the physical characteristics of helium.

_____

_____

33. List the pulmonary pathologies that may be treated with heliox therapy.

_____

_____

34. At what generation of the bronchi does turbulent flow transition to laminar flow?

_____

35. Calculate the actual flow reading for an 80:20 heliox mixture with a displayed flow rate of 6 L/min.

_____

_____

Chapter **23** **Special Techniques in Ventilatory Support**

36. Complete the following table, which compares volumes delivered during heliox therapy provided by critical care ventilators.

Ventilator	Volume with Heliox
CareFusion AVEA	_____
Hamilton Veolar and Galileo	_____
Puritan Bennett 7200	_____
Puritan Bennett 840	_____
Servo 300	_____
Servo^i	_____
Dräger Dura-2	_____
Dräger E4	_____

37. How is heliox connected to a mechanical ventilator?

_____

_____

38. How does the use of heliox with a mechanical ventilator affect F_IO_2 monitoring?

_____

_____

_____

_____

39. How does the use of heliox with a mechanical ventilator affect pressures?

_____

_____

40. Name a circumstance in which heliox therapy should not be used.

_____

_____

41. What is independent lung ventilation and how is it accomplished?

_____

_____

_____

42. List the surgical procedures in which lung isolation and ILV are used.

_____

_____

_____

43. Give two nonsurgical indications for ILV.

 a. _____

 b. _____

44. Compare synchronous with dyssynchronous ventilation when two ventilators are used for ILV.

_____

_____

_____

_____

_____

_____

45. Describe the procedure for measuring the lower inflection point and the upper inflection point using a slow-flow inflection point maneuver for each lung during ILV.

_____

_____

_____

_____

_____

_____

_____

_____

_____

46. Define *EIP*.

_____

_____

_____

47. What should the mode, rate, and V_T be for performing a less hemodynamically stressful slow-flow inflection maneuver to one lung? To both lungs?

_____

_____

48. How are appropriate levels of PEEP established for each lung during ILV?

_____

_____

_____

49. List the types of therapy that can be provided by the IPV-1 unit.

_____

_____

50. Describe the characteristics of the IPV-1 unit.

_____

_____

51. When administered with mechanical ventilation, how does the use of in-line IPV alter VC-CMV?

_____

_____

52. When administered with mechanical ventilation, how does the use of in-line IPV alter pressure controlled-continuous mandatory ventilation?

_____

_____

CRITICAL THINKING QUESTIONS

1. What ventilator mode and settings are represented by the following pressure-time graph?

_____

_____

2. After an adult patient is placed on HFOV, a chest radiograph shows the diaphragm in the midclavicular line to be at the level of the sixth posterior rib. Which ventilator parameter, if any, needs to be changed and why?

_____

_____

225

For questions 3 through 5, refer to the pressure-volume curve for a slow-flow inflection maneuver displayed in the following figure.

3. Plot the lower inflection point and the upper inflection point for the static pressure-volume loop.

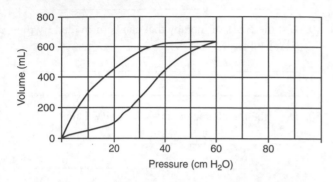

4. PEEP should be set at what level?

5. What V_T should be used to ventilate this patient?

CASE STUDIES

Case Study 1

A patient is ventilated with APRV at the following settings: P_{high} = 20 cm H_2O, P_{low} = 2 cm H_2O, T_{high} = 4 seconds, T_{low} = 1 second, F_IO_2 = 0.4. The patient's spontaneous rate is 12 breaths/min. The current ABG values include a PaO_2 of 86 mm Hg and a $PaCO_2$ of 68 mm Hg.

1. Calculate the current ventilator rate.

2. Which parameter needs to be changed to correct this patient's problem?

3. State the reason for changing that parameter.

Case Study 2

A patient currently is ventilated with APRV at the following settings: P_{high} = 35 cm H_2O, P_{low} = 5 cm H_2O, T_{high} = 7 seconds, T_{low} = 0.5 second, F_IO_2 = 0.3. The patient's spontaneous rate is 14 breaths/min. The current ABG values include a PaO_2 of 58 mm Hg and a $PaCO_2$ of 42 mm Hg.

1. Which parameter needs to be changed to correct this patient's problem?

2. State the reason for changing that parameter.

3. If changing the above parameter does not correct this patient's problem, what other change could be made?

Case Study 3

A male patient, 6 ft 2 in tall and weighing 81 kg, underwent thoracoabdominal surgical repair of an aortic aneurysm and has been brought to the SICU. He is intubated with a double lumen ET tube, and two ventilators are ready at the bedside.

1. Which lung will have sustained injury as a result of the surgery? Why?

2. What volume should be used in this patient to perform a single-lung slow inflation maneuver to determine inflection points?

3. If the right lung's lower inflection point is 6 cm H_2O and the left lung's lower inflection point is 18 cm H_2O, what is the appropriate PEEP level for each lung?

NBRC–STYLE QUESTIONS

1. The advantages of APRV over other forms of conventional ventilation are mainly the result of which of the following?
   a. Preservation of spontaneous breathing
   b. Reduced risk of ventilator-induced lung injury (VILI)
   c. Reduced risk of ventilator associated pneumonia (VAP)
   d. Reduced need for patient sedation and paralysis

2. Which of the following are the most appropriate APRV settings for an ARDS patient who is receiving VC-CMV at these settings: rate = 12 breaths/min, V_T = 600 mL, F_IO_2 = 1, PEEP = 10 cm H_2O, PIP = 32 cm H_2O, $P_{plateau}$ = 25 cm H_2O?
   a. P_{high} = 42 cm H_2O; P_{low} = 10 cm H_2O; T_{high} = 2 seconds; T_{low} = 2 seconds
   b. P_{high} = 25 cm H_2O; P_{low} = 10 cm H_2O; T_{high} = 4 seconds; T_{low} = 2 seconds
   c. P_{high} = 25 cm H_2O; P_{low} = 0; T_{high} = 4 seconds; T_{low} = 1 second
   d. P_{high} = 15 cm H_2O; P_{low} = 0; T_{high} = 6 seconds; T_{low} = 1.5 seconds

3. The parameter that can generally improve oxygenation during APRV is which of the following?
   a. P_{high}
   b. P_{low}
   c. T_{high}
   d. T_{low}

4. Calculate the APRV ventilator rate when T_{high} is 12 seconds and T_{low} is 2 seconds.
   a. 4 cycles/min
   b. 6 cycles/min
   c. 9 cycles/min
   d. 12 cycles/min

5. The first parameter set when starting HFOV is which of the following?
   a. $T_I\%$
   b. Frequency
   c. Amplitude
   d. Bias flow

6. A decrease in chest wiggle during HFOV may be caused by which of the following?
   1. Pneumothorax
   2. ET obstruction
   3. Increased $PaCO_2$
   4. Patient improvement
   a. 1 and 2
   b. 2 and 3
   c. 4
   d. 1 and 3

7. An ARDS patient is receiving HFOV at the following settings: P_{aw} = 28 cm H_2O, frequency = 6 Hz, bias flow = 30 L/min, ΔP = 7 (amplitude 60 cm H_2O), $T_I\%$ = 33, F_IO_2 = 0.8. The patient's PaO_2 on these settings is 75 mm Hg. Which of the following is the most appropriate action in this case?
   a. Increase the F_IO_2 to 0.9
   b. Reduce the control to 5
   c. Reduce the frequency to 5 Hz
   d. Increase the P_{aw} to 30 cm H_2O

8. With HFOV, the first step in reducing an adult patient's $PaCO_2$ is which of the following?
   a. Increase the $T_I\%$
   b. Reduce the frequency
   c. Increase the amplitude
   d. Increase the cuff leak

9. To achieve a flow of 8 L/min for a 70:30 heliox mixture, the oxygen flowmeter should be set at which of the following?
   a. 5 L/min
   b. 8 L/min
   c. 11 L/min
   d. 14 L/min

10. During ventilation with heliox mixtures, most ventilators have which of the following problems?
    1. Inaccurate PEEP measurements
    2. Discrepancies in flow measurements
    3. Discrepancies between the set and actual F_IO_2
    4. Nonlinear relationship between $V_T$set and $V_T$del
    a. 1 and 2
    b. 2 and 3
    c. 3 and 4
    d. 1 and 4

11. An adult patient has had a severe asthmatic episode and requires intubation. The most appropriate type of ventilation for this patient is which of the following?
    a. ILV
    b. APRV
    c. IPV
    d. PCV with heliox

12. An adult patient has a left-sided flail chest and underlying left lung contusions from a motor vehicle accident. The most appropriate type of ventilation for this patient is which of the following?
    a. ILV
    b. APRV
    c. HFOV
    d. PCV with heliox

13. With HFOV, volume delivery from the oscillator is determined by all of the following except:
    a. $T_I\%$
    b. Oscillator displacement
    c. ET tube size
    d. Patient's ability to trigger the ventilator

14. When heliox concentrations $\geq 50:50$ are used, the effect on the delivery of albuterol from an MDI during mechanical ventilation, as compared with the effects of oxygen or air, is which of the following?
    a. Delivery of albuterol is reduced by at least 25%.
    b. Delivery of albuterol is reduced by at least 50%.
    c. Delivery of albuterol is increased by at least 25%.
    d. Delivery of albuterol is increased by at least 50%.